VITAMIN POLITICS

VITAMIN POLITICS

by John Fried

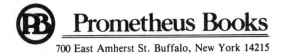

Prometheus Books

700 East Amherst St. Buffalo, New York 14215

For Eric Philip

Published 1984 by
Prometheus Books
700 East Amherst Street
Buffalo, New York 14215

ISBN 0-87975-222-X
Library of Congress Catalog Card No. 83-62187

Contents

Foreword

Vitamin. Like "vital" and "vitality," the very word suggests life itself. Today, more than seventy million Americans take vitamins regularly. Most think they are getting "insurance" against the possibility of a nutritional deficiency. Many also believe that high dosages of vitamins (megavitamins) prevent or are effective against disease.

Even more startling, over *one million* Americans are involved in *selling* vitamins through "health food" stores, pharmacies, supermarkets, mail order houses—and most significantly, huge multilevel sales companies like Shaklee, Amway, and Neo-Life.

Nutrition scientists call this situation a "vitamin craze." Ten years ago, John Fried decided to find out how it came about. Armed with a tape recorder, he traveled throughout the United States and Canada interviewing vitamin promoters and their critics. Concerned primarily about "megavitamin therapy," he was determined to answer two questions:

1. If the megavitamin proponents were right, why wouldn't the scientific community accept their beliefs?

2. If the scientists were correct, why hadn't they persuaded the public to ignore the proponents?

After sifting through mountains of data, Fried concluded that the megavitamin proponents were not only wrong, but they were more interested in publicity than scientific investigation. The completed study, published in 1975 by the Saturday Review Press as *The Vitamin Conspiracy,* was a classic. This 1984 edition is another.

Several things have changed in the interim. More studies have found that vitamin C does *not* prevent colds. Its proponents now claim that megadoses of vitamin C are effective against *cancer.* And when the FDA tried to regulate the sale of high dosage vitamins, promoters gained passage of a federal law to block this action. *Vitamin Politics* explores these topics and their implications for consumers.

If you take low doses of vitamins without advice from a qualified physician, this book may save you money. If you take megadoses or are thinking of doing so, this book might save your life. In any case, good citizens should know how vitamin politics has undermined laws designed to protect us all from harm.

Stephen Barrett, M.D.

Preface

La Vitamina Levanta Muertos
(Vitamins Raise The Dead)
Sign on a juice peddler's pushcart
in Puerto Vallarta, Mexico

As the 1960s melted into the 70s, vitamins were the hot topic of folk medicine.

Linus Pauling, the Nobel laureate, had become a public hero. The cure for the common cold had eluded the best efforts of the best minds in medicine. But it had not eluded him: Vitamin C, he told a world tired of coughing, sneezing, and hunting in the dark for the paper tissue box on the nightstand, was the simple and natural enemy of the cold. Evan and Wilfrid Shute, two Canadian physicians, had managed to convince millions that vitamin E could do what cardiologists, heart surgeons, and other medical experts could never hope to accomplish: end the ravages of heart disease. Dr. Abram Hoffer, a Canadian psychiatrist, had enticed a good many psychiatrists, psychologists, and other assorted healers of the psyche into believing that niacin and its chemical relatives could easily wipe away the ravages of mental illness. Adelle Davis (who was to die within a few years of cancer, a disease she had talked herself and others into hoping could be kept at bay with good nutrition) had converted a legion of followers to the cause of food worship, much of it revolving around vitamins.

As a journalist who had chosen to make medical reporting a specialty, I jumped with enthusiasm into an assignment to write a book about the field. Not just because there were so many fascinating characters among the provitamin forces, but because, it

9

seemed to me, conventional physicians and researchers were almost reduced to scientific impotence by the vitamin faddists.

Medical scientists had always been able to make some headway against quackery. It had been easy to prove that black boxes with blinking lights did not cure warts. Or that trips into gold mines did not banish arthritis. But no matter how hard they tried, nutritionists, doctors, and other health experts were unable to stem the tide of Americans intent on following the Pied Pipers of vitamins. I wanted to find out just why doctors and respectable nutritionists were failing.

In time I had my answers, and they resulted in the publication of the first version of this book, at the time titled *The Vitamin Conspiracy*. The book had its moment in the public eye. It was appropriately damned: Linus Pauling, upon receiving an advance copy, wrote the publisher and warned that in his eyes the book was "thoroughly unreliable . . . contains many erroneus statements." And, thankfully, it was praised. Geoffrey H. Bourne, editor of *World Review of Nutrition and Dietetics* and a leading authority in the field, said the assessments in the book were objective and that "the publishers will be doing the general public a favor by making this excellent report available to them."

In any case, I went on to other books and articles. In time, I imagined, vitamins would go the way of all American fads.

I was wrong.

As the 1970s wore on, the American passion for health and physical fitness grew more and more intense. More and more people took to jogging, running in marathons, swimming, biking, and working out in health gyms that were sprouting like mushrooms on the urban terrain. It was inevitable that, as part of this determination to stay healthy and young forever, millions of men and women would continue to turn to vitamins as added insurance against the possibility that they might age too quickly, develop heart disease, suffer a cold, fall into the melancholy of depression.

If anything, the mysticism surrounding vitamins thickened because some researchers were suddenly finding that some vitamins, given in large doses, could help some of their patients. Acne seemed to yield to a vitamin A derivative. Benign but troublesome breast lumps seemed to give way to vitamin E.

Perhaps more important, some researchers were suddenly taking seriously the possibility that some vitamins could play a limited role in the prevention of cancer.

And so when Dr. Stephen Barrett, probably the nation's most tireless anti-quackery campaigner, and Prometheus Books asked me to take another look at the vitamin field, I was glad to do so.

The book that is in your hands is the result of that second effort. It is, it should be noted, not so much a revision as an update. We have left much of the original book untouched, and it represents accurately the beliefs of the people who preached the value of vitamins all through the 1970s. While some of the enthusiasts may have changed their approach or may have moved onto other things, they have been supplanted by other players who have adopted the same philosophical approach as the one espoused by the people I talked with when I originally researched the book: Namely, that vitamins can be used as therapy for a host of human ills, major and minor. My revision job was greatly simplified precisely because so little had changed in the years since I had finished *The Vitamin Conspiracy.* In other words, the issues outlined in the original *Vitamin Conspiracy* are as valid today as they were in the mid-1970s.

One of the most important differences between this paperback edition and the original is that this version contains a full chapter on vitamins and cancer, whereas the original book contained only a two-page discussion of the topic. Other changes—that vitamin E is used with some success in fibrocystic disease of the breast, notations on deaths of some of the key figures in the vitamin field, some more material on the role of vitamin C in treating the common cold and other assorted tidbits—are, in effect, only addenda to the larger discussion.

In any case, my thanks go to Dr. Barrett for suggesting the update. I am also grateful to the following people for providing me with important research and information on vitamins: The National Cancer Institute/Office of Cancer Communications, Gordon Cohn and Armida Duran of the Kenneth Norris, Jr., Cancer Hospital and Research Institute at the University of Southern California, and Dr. A. L. Tappel of the University of California at Davis. A special measure of thanks is due to Dr.

Randy Cole. His doctorate is in computer science, not vitamins. But his help eased me through the often nerveracking task of learning to operate the word processor that made it possible for me to meet the publisher's deadline for this project.

CHAPTER I

Introduction

The fifteen to twenty white and brown bottles turn slowly as the lazy Susan standing on the low-slung coffee table winds down to an almost imperceptible turn. Larry Betzker, basking in the warm sunshine streaming in through the cathedral window in the high-ceilinged living room of the Spanish-style home in west Los Angeles, leans out of his easy chair, reaches out, and presses a finger to the moving tray's edge, braking it to a complete stop.

He scoops up one large bottle, opens it, and shakes an assortment of long, brown capsules into his hand. "We aren't all that systematic about it," he says, shaking the pills in his now closed hand like dice and continuing to explain why his family consumes up to fifty dollars' worth of vitamins and minerals a month. "The kids don't take them all the time, but we both take one and a half grams of C a day, a couple of thousand units of vitamin E, nicotinic acid, pyridoxine, B_{12}, well, everything in one way or another, I guess."

Betzker looks at his wife, Katherine, who is sitting on the edge of the couch and is leaning forward, her arms resting on her legs, her arms folded. "We both think they have helped us tremendously."

"Oh, absolutely," Katherine Betzker answers lightly. The house, the seven kids, her job as a university lecturer, she says, demand every bit of energy she can muster. "I can go sixteen hours a day and not feel it and I never get sick."

Katherine Betzker leans forward. Like her husband, she is in her late forties. She is a small, thin woman. Her black eyes are set in a small, sharply etched face. Her eyes, intense anyway, now grow even more serious. "And I'll tell you something else," she says conspiratorially, glancing at her husband, who is grinning because he senses what is coming. "Since Larry started on the vitamins, he has a hell of a lot more energy in bed too!"

Like millions of other Americans, the Betzkers have read book after book produced by vitamin evangelists, have read unquestioning articles in general circulation magazines (as well as those written for magazines whose sole purpose is to sell the compounds), have watched television shows which, in their hunger to entertain the bored housewife or the insomniac businessman, put on the air anyone who can weave an entrancing tale of medical magic. As a result, the Betzkers have been converted to the belief that vitamins in massive doses will protect them against scores of diseases and problems, including the ravages of old age, declining sex urges, receding energy, the onset of heart disease, the threat of mental illness, the bother of the common cold, the itch of dry skin, the frustration of sleeplessness, the specter of cancer, the aggravation of whining kids.

Nutritionists, doctors, and assorted researchers, horrified by the sight of people swallowing vitamin pill after vitamin pill, have tried to wage battle against the faddists who have conquered people like the Betzkers. These experts have gone to battle in part because they believe that much of the money spent on vitamins and other nutrients—estimated to be $3 billion every year—is flowing into the pockets of the very people who praise the vast health-giving potential of vitamins.

Dr. Stephen Barrett, chairman of the Lehigh Valley Committee Against Health Fraud, points out that *Prevention,* one of the leading magazines in the vitamin and nutrition fad world, is in essence a slick device that helps manufacturers of expensive vitamins and minerals hawk their wares. "You never see any claims made in ads in *Prevention* that this vitamin is good for this disease or that problem," Dr. Barrett says. "All the claims are made in editorial articles that surround the advertisements." This policy of touting inflated attributes for vitamins in editorial material rather than in the advertising, Barrett points out, has made

Prevention a tremendous financial success.

Prevention readers spend close to half a billion dollars a year on "food supplements," many of them advertised in the magazine. The average *Prevention* reader—the man or woman who is told in various articles of the miracles wrought by vitamins—spends hundreds of dollars a year on health products, many of them available from mail-order firms that advertise in *Prevention.*

Small wonder then that advertisements in *Prevention* tend to be expensive. A simple black and white full-page ad costs $15,047. A color page will set the advertiser back (very, very happily) $26,550. The advertiser who wants to put his ad on the highly visible back page of the magazine has to shell out $34,500 for a four-color ad. And yet, despite the high costs, the magazine, which tells its advertisers that they will reach 2.5 million readers, carries between sixty and one hundred pages of advertising each month.

The people that tout vitamins and the alleged benefits those vitamins have on health, in other words, are not motivated exclusively by the desire to help humanity.

"You have to remember that there is an economic factor in all of this," adds Dr. Leo Lutvak, a professor of medicine at the University of California at Los Angeles. "There are millions and millions of dollars going into the pockets of (the late) Adelle Davis and other food faddists. They are not doing this for altruistic reasons. They are after money. Adelle Davis's books (have sold) in the millions. The royalties she received from those books have been fantastic. She received royalties from health-food stores that sell preparations with her name on them. There are tie-in sales on all that stuff. There is a rip-off here."

As in any conflict, economic considerations are not the only factors that have led to the fighting. If nutrition experts have found it necessary to wage war against the vitamin enthusiasts, they have done so also because they have found their deepest philosophical feelings hurt.

Many of the nutritionists active in accepted vitamin research today are those who made early substantive inroads toward the understanding of vitamins. They have helped to isolate the various vitamins and came to understand that vitamins present in food help the body metabolize the food itself. They discovered that, in minute amounts, vitamins play specific roles in the functioning of body parts as diverse in form and function as the skin and eyes, that they help cells produce energy, that they participate in the building of genetic materials, and help form bones, red blood cells, and other tissues. All of these various functions, nutritionists feel, were ferreted out through judicious, painstaking, and time-consuming experimentation. So they resent—and have been compelled to fight—anyone who tries to prescribe farfetched uses for vitamins without taking the time and trouble to substantiate the hypothesis upon which the recommendation is based.

Thus the greatest wrath and the most searing attacks are reserved for those vitamin faddists who are deserters, the defectors from the ranks of reason—meaning the ranks of organized medicine and accepted scientific research protocol—who have chosen to fight with the faddists. When it comes to conversations about Linus Pauling or the Doctors Shute (two Canadian physicians who have been the prime champions of vitamin E) many "establishment" researchers verge on the apoplectic.

I asked Professor Thomas Jukes, a nutrition expert at the University of California at Berkeley, how he feels about the claims made for vitamin C. Jukes scurries over to a bookcase and fishes out Pauling's *Vitamin C and the Common Cold.* In case you haven't read Professor Pauling's book, you should know that he gives a great deal of credit to a Dr. Irwin Stone, a chemist, for putting him on the trail of vitamin C. "In April 1966, I received a letter from Dr. Irwin Stone, a biochemist whom I had met at the Carl Neuberg Medal Award Dinner in New York the previous month," Pauling writes in the introduction to his book. "He mentioned in his letter that I had expressed a desire to live for the next fifteen or twenty years. He said that he would like to see me remain in good health for the next *fifty* years, and that he was accordingly sending me a description of his high-level ascorbic acid regime. . . ." Jukes, bristling with rising indignation, struggling to control the fury in his voice, his angry eyes darting over the page, reads the appropriate passage. "This man Stone is a brewing chemist. He worked for Wallenstein out on Long Island."

Jukes slams shut the heavy reference book. "He writes Pauling and says, 'Dear Dr. Pauling, I hope you live forever.' Remember the salutation the king used to get, 'O King, live forever'? So Pauling thinks, say, this is great. So he went on this vitamin C kick.

"I heard recently that he couldn't attend a meeting of the AMA because he was home with a cold. Did you hear that?"

No, I hadn't heard that. Struck by Jukes's vehemence, I suddenly find myself playing devil's advocate. But Pauling is a respectable scientist, I say. Shouldn't he know, shouldn't he be able to judge if something were helping him? "A typical example of psychological healing. Psychological medicine."

But Pauling is a Nobel laureate in chemistry, an eminent and respected scientist! "Pauling is a past master of salesmanship. How do you think he got two Nobel Prizes? [1] By selling himself. There are a lot of people in chemistry who deserve the Nobel Prize, but only a few get it. The ones who get it not only have to be great scientists but have to be showmen. They work at it.

"A lot of these stories get started with someone like Professor Pauling. He didn't get colds for a few weeks when he took a lot of ascorbic acid, so the idea gets fixed in his mind and the rest of the time he spends trying to prove a preconceived notion. That is not the way to do research. That is what Shute is up to. He's got a thing about vitamin E. Vitamin E all the time."

Speaking of vitamin E: the Doctors Shute—brothers Wilfrid and Evan—have been claiming for more than a quarter of a century now that vitamin E is an effective agent to be used against all sorts of heart problems, that it helps the heart stave off the effects of diseases ranging from angina pectoris to rheumatic fever. The Shutes say they have treated thousands of patients successfully with vitamin E, that experiments around the world have proven the worth of the vitamin in treating heart disease, gangrene, and burns. Could it be, I ask, just for the sake of argument, that the Shutes, because they are sitting in a small, remote city in Canada, are being ignored because they are not in the mainstream of medicine, because they are small country doctors and are not attached to some major research institution?

For a moment there, I think Jukes is going to throttle me. But instead he bounds across the room, sweeps a framed photograph off a shelf and pushes it to my nose. "Speaking of the small country doctor," he spits, virtually talking through his teeth now, jabbing a

---

[1] In Chemistry and for his efforts in behalf of Peace.

finger at a man in the photograph. "There is one. That man had a medical practice in a small town in Ontario about sixty miles north of Toronto. He was a failure. He sold his practice. He sold his books. He went to the University of Toronto and asked for laboratory space, and a professor gave it to him. He asked for money to buy experimental dogs. He had a total budget of a hundred dollars. What do you think he did with it? He discovered insulin." The man was Dr. Frederick Banting. And he discovered insulin because he conducted well-thought-out experiments with laboratory animals, experiments that proved the worthiness of a theory he had, and tested and retested a substance that had been born of that idea before it was unleashed on the public. Jukes takes another slap with the back of his hand at the picture he has been holding. I hadn't noticed the dog in the photograph before. "That is the first dog to be kept alive with insulin," Jukes says. "Did the medical profession turn down insulin? No! The medical profession doesn't turn down great discoveries so long as they work."

Jukes returns his prized photograph to its place on the shelf and turns to face me once more. Now he looks sad. The anger has drained from him. "To think of all these wonderful discoveries made with vitamins, how they lifted the burden of vitamin deficiencies from the world and then have it degenerate into . . . this hucksterism . . . It's disappointed me."

Conventional doctors, nutritionists, and biochemists have been deeply frustrated in battles against the vitamin enthusiasts. "You are dealing essentially with fanatics, and food is their religion," says Dr. Bernard T. Kaufman, chief of the Vitamin Metabolism Section at the National Institutes of Health in Bethesda, Maryland. That means, of course, that the nutrition scientist can no more convince the nutrition religionist and his would-be followers of the errors in their thinking than the evolution expert can convince a fundamentalist Baptist preacher and his congregation of the folly of the belief that man is a direct descendant of a piece of mud fashioned by a God lonely for a little companionship.

Not only are the vitamin faddists like religious fanatics, but they have, like all ardent believers, become masters of the specious argument. Against all this, the conventional scientist really has no effective weapons. "These people are extremely glib," says Dr.

Kaufman. "They can talk you into anything. You can come down with your reams of data and they'll talk you right out of them. They'll show that you are a liar, a fraud, and a communist."

(Kaufman is not engaging in hyperbole. For more than ten years the Food and Drug Administration, in its own bureaucratic fashion, tried to bring the vitamin industry under control, to rein in the overenthusiastic claims made for vitamins and to put a damper on the thrust toward selling the public ever more potent, ever more expensive vitamin combinations. Commented Gary Allen, a crusading anticommunist in the September, 1973, issue of *American Opinion,* an ultraconservative magazine: "Operating on Washington's usual dictum that the public doesn't know what is best for itself, the moguls of F.D.A. don't claim that vitamins or health foods are toxic and otherwise harmful. You see, they just don't want you to waste your money, and if Big Brother can force you to stop wasting your cash on 'frivolous' vitamins and nutrition he will have established a precedent for deciding how you will spend the rest of your income which survives his tax collectors.")

Faced by their inability to win the hearts and minds of the public at large and to convince them that the vitamin faddists are wrong, nutritional experts have been forced to carry out hit and run attacks against their enemies. In large part, these attacks have consisted of thrusts and parries in the forms of outraged personal protests to some of the more visible targets in the vitamin-fad trenches, namely, leaders of the opposition forces like Adelle Davis. One physician protested that Miss Davis was causing many parents a good deal of pain by warning that babies denied breast feeding were particularly prone to the Sudden Infant Death Syndrome (also known as crib death) and that a good supply of vitamin E and better nutrition might prevent such deaths. SIDS, Miss Davis was told, had never been linked to any particular feeding patterns, and breast-fed babies, it was pointed out to her, were no less likely to fall prey to the mysterious syndrome. "Thank you so much for correcting me," Miss Davis wrote the physician. "It was the first time I had heard that such crib deaths occur in infants while they are being breast fed. I am indeed sorry if words of mine have added to the suffering of parents whose infants have died."

In much the same way, a group of nutrition experts succeeded in luring Miss Davis to a luncheon in Washington, D.C., back in the spring of 1973. During the luncheon, the participants peppered Miss Davis with inconsistencies and mistakes they had culled from her books. Why, one doctor wanted to know, did Miss Davis advocate massive doses of vitamin A for children when it was well known that vitamin A poisoning brought on symptoms similar to those produced by brain tumors? Miss Davis listened and replied that she would accept the "criticism and will watch carefully and take it seriously." Other questions brought similar answers. But none of these admonitions or admissions of error, as the participants in this luncheon knew, could be counted as significant battle victories for the forces of reason. "The trouble with her corrections," Dr. Edward H. Rynearson, emeritus professor of medicine at the Mayo Clinic, noted, "was that they never had the impact of her vociferous presentations; a confused public remains confused."

More often than not, establishment researchers do not get a chance to engage in hand-to-hand combat with the vitamin faddists. As a result, they are reduced to an even more ineffectual ploy—sitting around the campfire, pointing out to each other weaknesses in the beliefs espoused by their opponents. Thus, Dr. Rynearson, Dr. Roslyn Alfin-Slater, an eminent nutritionist at the University of California at Los Angeles, and Dr. George V. Mann, professor of biochemistry and medicine at Vanderbilt University, have sifted through Adelle Davis's books extensively and have written to each other about her many mistakes—though none of this knowledge has ever been fashioned into an effective weapon to use against Davis.

When Adelle Davis was invited to speak (over the strenuous and stormy protests of many nutrition experts) at the University of California Alumni Centennial in 1973, nutritionists and vitamin researchers were reduced to passing around a printed version of her speech, underlining what they considered to be its worst errors. "She made seventeen errors," Dr. Gladys Emerson of the UCLA School of Public Health told me. "She said you can't get vitamin D in food, and vitamin D is available in liver. She said that eggs are a good source of calcium. They are, if you eat the shells. There is virtually no calcium in the egg itself. She said that the B vitamins are hard to get. They are not. In California, the enrichment of flour with vitamin B is mandatory. B_1, B_{12}, nicotinic acid are all required in enrichment programs in the southern states."

To a large extent, nutritional and vitamin experts say, they have been unable to hold their own in battles with the faddists because the public is far more interested in romantic hogwash than scientific truth. "When Adelle Davis would get on the radio and start talking about the miraculous cures with vitamin E, that her cleaning woman's son was working in a car wash, was scalded by steam and all the skin came off his back, and she put vitamin E on it and two weeks later he was playing football, that's the kind of talk people listen to," Professor Jukes laments. "If someone gets up and says it took ten years of research before any need for vitamin E in human beings was determined and that no one has been able to show that [a vitamin E deficiency] occurs spontaneously but can only be reproduced in an artificial diet, no one listens to it.

"The facts of science are so cold, so uninteresting and dry. It's the magical stories that catch the public eye."

Jukes is absolutely right. Among the vitamin enthusiasts, the most potent weapon that might be used in annihilating opposition is the anecdote, the wondrous story of the way a vitamin has helped a hapless human being return to a normal life. The anecdotal evidence is propagated not just by the professionals who have come to believe devoutly in vitamins but by laymen who have taken to experimenting with them as well.

For example: according to a man we'll call Corley, his efforts against mental illness were losing battles until he discovered megavitamins. In 1967, Corley relates, he was hospitalized in a mental hospital three times. When he was not an inpatient at the hospital, he was seeing a psychiatrist once a week. And through it all he was on heavy doses of tranquilizers and antidepressants, including Thorazine, Mellaril, and Impramine. "The drugs and disease kept me in what can be best defined as limbo," Corley relates. "After eighteen months of this, I went to a Schizophrenics Anonymous meeting. There I learned about the megavitamin therapy."

Corley had gone to the meeting because he felt he had reason to believe that he was a schizophrenic. The talk that vitamins—particularly nicotinic acid—could control the disease excited Corley.

He bought himself vitamins and began to treat himself. "The vitamins did help me," he says. "For the first time in my life I did not go to bed tired and get up more tired than when I went to bed. The reduction in fatigue was the best improvement. I also felt less fearful and anxious than I had. I stopped taking the Mellaril and Tofranil."

Anecdotes such as this one do not constitute scientific proof. Cautious scientific investigators know that neither patients who take a new medicine or drug nor those who advocate its use can be objective about the results it elicits. Individual case histories, furthermore, mean nothing in evaluating the overall efficacy of a drug. Some people do not react to any drug. Would it have been wise to ban aspirin because people here and there (even hundreds of people) had sworn that they received no relief for their headaches by taking the drug? Thalidomide proved to be a devastatingly dangerous drug. Would it have been acceptable to go on prescribing the drug for pregnant women because a few swore it helped them and because those women did not bear deformed children? In the enthusiasm for any new agent, breathless descriptions of its alleged good effects often obscure the anecdotes that might tell of its darker sides.

Because any new compound can have good and bad effects and because researchers know that a high number of patients will react in positive fashion to anything they are given, new drugs are usually studied by double-blind methods. A group of people who have the illness the new drug should cure or alleviate is divided in half. Half the group gets the experimental drug. The other half receives an inert preparation, a placebo. Neither the patients participating in the experiment nor the doctors assessing their progress know who is getting what. Drug and placebo are passed out in bottles marked with a code. At the end of the experiment the code is broken, and the changes in the patients are collated and studied statistically. Since many patients given a placebo will show a positive reaction, the new substance has to elicit results that are significantly better than those elicited by the placebo in order to be seriously considered for admission into the official drug armamentarium. For example, if 15 percent of the people in a group of patients receiving a placebo say they feel better after taking the inert substance, perhaps 25 or 30 percent (the statistician and the researchers actually decide what percentage is considered significant) in the other group, the group receiving the new drug, would have to show positive results in order for the researchers to take the drug seriously.

Aware that their evidence is sometimes suspect, vitamin faddists often skirt the issue by purporting to report scientific studies that allegedly support their enthusiasm for vitamin therapies.

Research Publications in Sunnyvale, California, is an organization that keeps track of "advances" in research with vitamin C. Research Publications, among other things, prints and distributes a "data" sheet that reports and abstracts advances that might be encouraging to people worried about an assortment of human ills, including cancer and heart disease.

Read superficially, the "data" sheet—entitled *New Information and Recent Findings Concerning Vitamin C*—appears to be a concise compendium of hundreds of experiments and research studies into the properties and possibilities of vitamin C. There seems to be little reason to question the information that is presented. Only when the references accompanying the various reports are checked does the rosy picture of vitamin C begin to wilt somewhat.

New Information and Recent Findings Concerning Vitamin C implies that many of the findings it reports were discovered by different researchers carrying on independent studies. For example, three different and separate items in the newsletter read: "Vitamin C apparently flushes deposits of cholesterol out of arteries. Long term vit [*sic*] C deficiency causes plaques of cholesterol to form on artery walls which are eventually dissolved with a prolonged program of increased vit C (*Lancet,* Dec. 1971, p. 1280). . . . There is strong supporting evidence to conclude that the lack of vit C is the only factor involved in the cause of atherosclerosis (*Lancet,* April 8, 1972). . . . Vit C is essential for the proper metabolism of fats. If the balance between C and fats favors C, the fats will always be properly metabolized (broken down), and the arteries will remain clean (*Lancet,* Oct. 31, 1970)."

Nowhere in the data sheet is there a clue that these three "findings" are in fact not new discoveries but the opinions of one person, Dr. Constance Spittle, a British physician, whose views are based partly on a few of her own observations and research but mostly on her interpretation of studies conducted by others. (Nowhere, moreover, is there a clue that most of Dr. Spittle's views are contained not in articles in *Lancet,* the prestigious British medical journal, but in letters to the editor, a highly informal method of communication in the hierarchy of scientific reportage.)

On delving further, it is obvious, too, that Dr. Spittle is not very painstaking in accurately interpreting the work conducted by these other scientists. In one of her letters to *Lancet,* a letter cited by Research Publications, Dr. Spittle tells the journal's readers that there is "very strong supportive evidence" that vitamin C is the only factor involved in the development of atherosclerotic disease.

In her letter Dr. Spittle cites a number of theories for her own ideas on the subject and then goes on to say that one study, conducted in Scotland, backs up the vitamin C–atherosclerosis link. That study, she writes, demonstrated that deaths from heart attacks have a seasonal variation and that this variation could be correlated with maximum and minimum intakes of vitamin C. Heart-attack deaths are at their highest peaks when there is little vitamin C available (during and just after the winter) and at their lowest peaks when there have been plenty of vitamin-C-bearing fruits around, namely, toward the end of summer.

The original Scottish study did in fact find that there is a seasonal variation in deaths from heart attacks in the British Isles. But in citing the study Dr. Spittle conveniently forgot to mention some of the other conclusions the Scottish researchers had reached. If heart attacks are at their highest in spring—a time when fruits are not yet fully available and the population has gone through several months of relative vitamin C deprivation—one reason might be, the Scots had said, that blood pressure, a considerable risk factor in heart disease, also seems to reach high peaks in spring. The authors also noted (and Spittle and Research Publications did not) that in their research they found that there was a comparable rise in *all* causes of death during the winter and early-spring months. The Scottish researchers, who had mentioned the shortages of vitamin C only in passing, also speculated on other reasons behind the seasonal fluctuation in deaths from heart attacks. "It may be a direct cause and effect relationship or it may reflect indirectly seasonal variation in the incidence of infection," they suggested. "Experimental observations on rats suggest that cold exposure can cause increased ventricular [the ventricle is the main pumping chamber of the heart] work and excitability, perhaps because of increased thyroidal activity. It is therefore possible that cold exposure increases the severity of damage to the myocardium [the muscle of the heart]. . . ." Spittle's abbreviated report of the Scottish study never comes across to the reader of *New Information* who, anxious about his own problems with heart disease, runs out to buy carloads of vitamin C to help him rid himself of his atherosclerosis.

Linus Pauling, the Shutes, Dr. Abram Hoffer in Canada (he believes that vitamins in massive doses can control schizophrenia), Adelle Davis, have all recommended their regimens because they believe that theoretically there is no reason why their ideas should not work. Investigations by leading medical researchers have not proved their theories. They have no conclusive body of proof: there are enough bits and pieces of information, they believe, to warrant the practice of what might be called theoretical medicine. This tendency to believe that their theories can only be right and can only lead to good would not be disturbing if vitamins given in massive doses were, at worst, ineffective. But vitamins given in vast quantities are, strickly speaking, no longer vitamins. They are drugs. And like many drugs they can have, and do have, dangerous side effects.

Children seem to be particularly vulnerable to vitamin poisonings, especially when they are under the care of parents who adhere much too enthusiastically to Adelle Davis. According to one San Francisco physician, Dr. John C. Bolton, a woman who had been raising her children according to Adelle Davis's *Let's Have Healthy Children* was forced to bring her four-year-old daughter to the University of California Medical Center in San Francisco because the girl appeared to be seriously ill. The child had had a four-month history of repeated episodes of vomiting, diarrhea, dehydration, irritability, and fever. Doctors suspected hyperparathyroidism and were weighing the possibility of removing the girl's parathyroid gland. Further investigations disclosed that the mother had been feeding the girl up to 100,000 units of vitamin A a day, as well as astronomical amounts of other vitamins and minerals. When the vitamins were discontinued, the child returned to normal.

Doctors at Yale University's School of Medicine treated two children—a brother and sister—brought to the hospital with vitamin poisoning. The children's mother, who did not believe in immunization, had been giving the children massive doses of vitamins for a year, believing they would protect the children against disease. The girl had been brought into the hospital because she had begun to be irritable and had started to vomit almost constantly. A thorough examination revealed that her head was growing abnormally because her skull bones had begun to enlarge. When the mother stopped giving the child vitamin A (she had been taking 25,000 international units a day for a year), the symptoms stopped and her head size returned to normal. The girl's brother, thirty months old, was also treated at the hospital because he had grown lethargic and was unable to walk because he had severe pain in both shins. A medical examination showed he was missing patches of hair on his head, that his liver and spleen were enlarged, and that his skull bones, too, had grown abnormally. He had been getting 57,000 international units of vitamin A, 1,000 international units of D, 2,000 international units of E, 480 milligrams of ascorbic acid, 1,600 milligrams of calcium, and 750 milligrams of phosphate a day. When the vitamins were stopped, his problems disappeared and his skull slowly returned to its normal size.

The mighty forces of the federal bureaucracy have also tried to rout the vitamin enthusiasts and bring the war to an end. But even at a time when they have been able to bring major environmental polluters to account, the makers of rules and regulations have failed in their efforts to bring vitamin adherents to heel.

The Food and Drug Administration, for example, tried as far back as 1962 to promulgate some sensible guidelines for the sale and advertising of vitamins. But the agency had hardly written its recommendations before vitamin adherents trained their sights on its buildings in Washington. Over the next decade, the FDA was forced to hold protracted discussion and debates, to defend itself against a continuous procession of lawsuits, and to hold formal hearings that lasted two years, a process that yielded little more than thirty-two thousand pages of transcripts that were soon gathering dust on a long bookshelf in the FDA's building in a Maryland suburb of Washington, D.C.

The fight against the FDA even went to Congress. One bill, commonly known as H.R. 643, was introduced by former

California Republican Representative Craig Hosmer. Hosmer's district included the home of the National Health Federation, a group heavily involved in a number of questionable ventures (according to the American Medical Association, the group's members have repeatedly run afoul of the law for trying to sell worthless medicines and cure-all gadgets), and now a fervent champion of vitamin therapies and other so-called alternative medicines.

The bill, in its original form, would have forbidden the FDA from exercising any power in the control of vitamins, and many of Hosmer's colleagues agreed to cosponsor the bill out of courtesy or to gain his support for their own pet bills. However, when a *New York Times* reporter, Richard D. Lyons, began to make inquiries into Hosmer's efforts to hamstring the FDA, a good many people on Capitol Hill found themselves thoroughly embarrassed. "Thousands of food faddists, 142 Congressmen, and a health lobby, which the Federal Government has linked to quackery, are backing an obscure bill . . ." Lyons wrote in the May 14, 1973, issue of the *Times*. ". . . Some of the co-sponsoring Congressmen appear not to have the foggiest notion of the contents of H.R. 643 which would lift Federal controls on dosages and sales of vitamins."

No matter. At one time or another, the number of Congressmen willing to sponsor legislation to get the FDA off the back of the vitamin enthusiasts ran to 240. The Senate was no less judicious in its approach: eighty-three Senators at one point went on record favoring the moves to cut the FDA out of the vitamin field.

When Senator William Proxmire, a Democrat from Wisconsin, entered the arena, however, the FDA's efforts to bring vitamin hucksterism under control were doomed. Proxmire, who is almost as fanatic about controlling the federal bureaucracy as he is about staying in shape, sponsored, with the help of Senator Richard Schweiker, his own provitamin, anti-FDA bill. It was a piece of legislation *Consumer Reports* predicted would, among other things "inevitably invite irrational fortification (of foods with vitamins) solely for promotional purposes." Perhaps even more deplorable, *Consumer Reports* said in June 1973, Proxmire's bill would "reverse the trend of Federal law since 1938 requiring manufacturers to prove a product safe before it is marketed. It would require the FDA to prove a vitamin or mineral preparation *unsafe (CR's* emphasis) before limiting its sale, an immensely difficult task."

The Proxmire-Schweiker bill passed. But the battle didn't stop there. Early in 1979, the FDA tried to wiggle out from under the restrictions imposed on it by Congress and announced new proposals that would have treated vitamins (and minerals) as over-the-counter drugs. Once again, the provitamin forces went into action and soon Senators and Congressmen were receiving outraged (and outrageous) letters and postcards from their constituents angry over the FDA's refusal to allow them their beloved vitamins.

As a partial response, Senators Orrin Hatch of Utah and S. I. Hayakawa of California sponsored the "Voluntary Vitamin Act of 1981." It would have eviscerated all FDA attempts to control the unfettered use of vitamins. The bill obviously angered those already unhappy with what they considered to be the excessive vitamin consumption taking place in the United States. "In drugstores, supermarkets, health-food stores, and by door-to-door salesmen, we are incessantly confronted with vitamins," Dr. Jukes argued in an article in a 1982 issue of the *Journal of Nutrition Education.* "American urine is the richest in the world. No 'Voluntary Vitamins Act' is needed. Unregulated vitamins are figuratively coming out of our ears."

(Jukes's remark that American urine is the richest in the world was a whimsical reference to the fact that most vitamins are water soluble and that once the body is saturated with these vitamins whatever additional doses are taken are soon excreted in the urine. Thus, one argument against the consumption of megadoses of vitamin C is that the body is filled with all the vitamin C it can store after only a relatively small amount has been ingested. The body gets rid of the rest.)

Before Congress could act on Hatch's bill, a new Food and Drug administrator, Arthur Hull Hayes, was appointed. He backed off the newly proposed FDA regulations. As a result, momentum for the Hatch bill petered out. The FDA withdrew from the field once again to lick its wounds.

One suspects that the war, whether it engages only respectable authorities and the quacks or whether it draws in, from time to time, various governmental agencies, will not end with a decisive victory for any side. Rather, it may very well become a war of attrition, one in which the food faddists will happily go on fighting for their mythical visions of vitamins while a handful of anti-quackery crusaders will try to stop them. The bulk of the establishment researchers, disgusted by their inability to convince the public that illness has no magical cures and that mortality, whether we like it or not, is the inevitable lot of every human being, will simply drop their efforts and return to their laboratories. There at least, they will have to face only the peculiarities of human chemistry and human biology, matters far less puzzling than human nature.

(Some scientists are not happy that many of their colleagues refuse to do battle with the vitamin nuts. "We have shrugged off rather than rejected forcefully the cultists, the misfits, and the fools who erode science," Nobel laureate Arthur Kornberg told the *Peninsula Times Tribune* in Oakland, California, recently. "Society, by ignorance, is as captive to creationists, astrologers, evangelists, food faddists, and all kinds of gurus as were our ancestors by fears of thunder and lightning.")

In researching the medical literature and in talking to dozens of experts, I became convinced, after starting out more or less neutral on the matter, that vitamins in massive doses are of no value to 99.9 percent of the people swallowing them. The other 0.1 percent has a legitimate need for hundreds and thousands of milligrams of various vitamins and should be under the care of a qualified physician with expert knowledge of vitamin metabolism problems.

Anyone who makes a careful study of the claims made for vitamins has to be impressed by a curious fact. Many of the diseases and problems—major and minor—said to be curable or controllable by massive infusions of vitamins are diseases in which the subjective judgment of the patient and the enthusiastic vitamin prescriber plays an important role in evaluating the course of the condition. Many of the problems are those with a history that is highly irregular and subject to change for no apparent reason. Most diseases or discomforts are self-limiting and tend to end in time, no matter what anyone does. In other words it becomes apparent that vitamin enthusiasts are touting vitamins for diseases whose disappearance or amelioration could just as well be correlated with a patient's habit of snapping his fingers as with his devout dedication to the swallowing of dozens of vitamin pills a day.

CHAPTER II

Vitamins and Cancer

Cancer is a disease that looms large in our lives. Many of us have watched a parent, a child, a sibling, a grandparent struggle with the disease. Many of us have made the emotionally laden pilgrimages to the bedside of a gaunt, fear-ridden, semiconscious friend who was once a vital, active human being. Not a few of us have quietly listened to the last benedictions said over the coffin containing the body of a colleague who has finally lost the struggle against the disease.

Cancer, moreover, is not a disease that strikes only at others. Thus, it looms large because it seems to most of us that there is little we can do to escape its deadly grip. We can stop smoking and lower the odds that we'll develop cancer of the lung, mouth, or throat. And maybe, if some experts are right, we can lower the fat content of our diets and reduce our risk of contracting cancer of the colon, bladder, or breast. But beyond that what can we do? We can't always stop breathing polluted air, quit jobs that expose us to carcinogens, move out of homes riddled with asbestos, or leave areas where toxic wastes may have infiltrated the soil.

Although medical science has made important strides in controlling some cancers and even curing a few, the disease retains its ability to frighten because, to many people, the modes of treatment seem even worse than the malignancy itself. Surgery, radiation, and therapy with highly poisonous chemicals offer a chance at life, though at an often terrible price.

Because there are few among us who do not dread this vicious illness, it is hardly surprising that it has caught the eye of faddists who believe that vitamins can cure anything. Dr. William Jarvis, a prominent California anti-quackery crusader, summarizes it well: "It would be hard to find a disease better designed for the needs of quackery than cancer. Fear causes people to act irrationally and cancer victims not only feel fear, but guilt, rejection, and inner revulsion to a far greater extent than do victims of other life-threatening disease."

At the same time, it is not particularly astonishing that the medical establishment, which for the better part of two decades has been trying to convince the public that vitamins are not a panacea, is now desperately trying to combat the belief that vitamin C (among others) will not grant us a reprieve from the scourge of cancer. But in this struggle, the efforts of the medical establishment are tinged with a special irony: While some doctors and anti-quackery experts have been warning that the faith in the anti-cancer potential of vitamins has been exaggerated, a number of cancer researchers have been finding tantalizing clues that vitamins, perhaps even the vitamin content of our diets, may play an important role in the control of some forms of cancer.

The vitamin treatments offered up as simple cures for cancer have been many and varied.

Dr. Harold Manner, a former researcher in developmental biology at Loyola University in Chicago, gave up academia to dedicate himself to the Metabolic Research Foundation in Glenview, Illinois. From there, Manner has put out the word that cancer can indeed be conquered with changes in nutritional habits. Manner's "metabolic program" includes the use of "natural foods," a diet that supposedly requires the body to use less of its energy to digest food. It also encourages the use of coffee enemas, fasting, and, of course, vitamins. In West Germany, meanwhile, Dr. Hans Hoefer-Janker treats cancer patients with radiation and chemotherapy—and a mixture concocted from enzymes and a vitamin A solution.

American Cancer Society experts have reviewed Manner's work and have found it "grossly . . . unsound and unscientific." Hoefer-Janker's work has fared no better with careful investigators, who have reported that he uses excessive amounts of a chemotherapy drug that can cause bladder injury. According to the National Cancer Institute, Hoefer-Janker's "data on . . . enzymes and (vitamin A solution) have been reviewed in the United States, but as yet remain unproven therapies against cancer."

One very shady practitioner, working out of Grapevine, Texas, has had his own, very dubious ideas about cancer. Among other things, this man was convinced that 83 percent of all cancer in the United States could be eliminated if people would just stop eating protein after 1 o'clock in the afternoon. Those who had not watched their afternoon intake of proteins, this pseudo-scientist said, had paid the price by developing severe shortages of pancreatic enzymes and, as a result, cancer. Until the courts finally put him out of business, the Grapevine man told those unfortunate cancer patients who had come to him in their desperate search for a cure that their hope lay in a "perfectly balanced co-enzyme-vitamin-mineral compound . . . concentrated vitamin formula of C, bioflavonoids, and rutin" and a host of other nutrients.

Although many vitamin practitioners (legitimate researchers who have gone astray as well as the out-and-out quacks) who preach the efficacy of vitamins as anti-cancer compounds have been relatively easy to dismiss, other enthusiasts have not. One of them is Linus Pauling.

In the mid-1970s Pauling and a Scottish researcher, Ewan Cameron of Vale of Leven District General Hospital in Loch Lomondside, reported on 100 terminal and "untreatable" cancer patients who had been treated with massive doses of vitamin C. The patients lived somewhat longer than a group of 1,000 terminal patients who had not received C, Pauling and Cameron said. Moreover, the patients had reported less pain than other patients. In a few cases, the two researchers added, there had even been a measurable regression of the malignant tumor.

Many experts viewed Pauling and Cameron's ideas with a good deal of skepticism, particularly because the two had not used sound scientific methods to reach their conclusions. Pauling and Cameron said that they had taken care to make sure that patients in the two groups had been matched for age, sex, and location and type of cancer. However, some critics pointed out, Pauling and Cameron had given no indication that this matching—crucial to insure that like situations were being compared—had been carried out within specific subgroups. That is, Pauling and Cameron may have insured that there were the same number of fifty-five-year-olds among the 100 people treated with C as there had been among the 1,000 not treated with C. But seemingly they did not see to it, for example, that the colon cancer patients who received C were about the same age as the colon cancer victims not given the vitamin. Nor was there evidence that Pauling and Cameron had insured that they compared patients by weight, by the sites to which their cancers had spread, etc.

Perhaps more important, the critics said, was the definition of the term "untreatable." Cameron, the doubters said, maintained that he started his patients on vitamin C when he thought they would not be treatable by other methods. A case that may have been "untreatable" to Cameron, may not have appeared that way to another physician. In fact, by studying some of Cameron and Pauling's statistics, researchers noted that colon cancer patients given vitamin C had been diagnosed as "untreatable" after they had been under Cameron's care for an average of 106 days. But the colon cancer patients with whom they had been compared had been followed for 283 days before they had been given the "untreatable" designation. According to Dr. William D. Dewys, chief of the clinical investigations branch at the National Cancer Institute's Cancer Therapy Program, "Cameron's patients would be expected to have less advanced disease and a better remaining life expectancy than would the control patients. Thus, their survival would have been expected to be better—regardless of what treatment they were given."

Faced by these objections, Pauling and Cameron went back to their records. They found that some of the patients among those who had not received vitamin C should not have been included in their study because those patients had not be properly evaluated. They substituted other patients whose prognoses and conditions had been checked more thoroughly. But even when after these adjustment had been made and the data reexamined, Pauling and Cameron reported, there was no reason for them to change their minds about the efficacy of vitamin C. "Our conclusion is that the results previously reported are valid," Cameron and Pauling wrote in the *Proceedings of the National Academy of Science* in 1978. "In fact, the increase in life expectancy of ascorbate-treated patients with terminal cancer is found to be somewhat larger than we previously reported."

The doubters were not convinced. In an editorial following the Pauling and Cameron reassessment, Dr. Julius H. Comroe, Jr., a member of the *Proceedings'* editorial board, pointed out that Pauling and Cameron had presented "no new ideas, concepts or approaches" and that they "have not used well-established rules for clinical investigation to support their thesis."

Though Pauling and Cameron had failed to convince the scientific community that vitamin C could be a potent anti-cancer weapon, they had gained a sympathetic, if not downright eager, audience among lay people. And because public acceptance of their claims was so strong, researchers at the Mayo Clinic in Rochester decided to test vitamin C according to the precepts accepted by conventional medical researchers.

The Mayo researchers were willing to entertain the notion that C could help in the fight against cancer because lymphocytes, cells that help the body's immune system fight disease, are rich in vitamin C. The Mayo people also knew that when mice are given high doses of vitamin C their immune systems are better able to fight off disease. Moreover, the group knew, in some humans some cell changes that lead to cancer seem to give way to doses of vitamin C.

For their study, the Mayo researchers chose 150 patients with highly advanced cancer and divided them into two groups. Patients in one group received 10 grams of vitamin C. The patients in the other group received a pill made to taste like C. Other than that, the groups were made up of men and women who were very much alike in age, in the area where their cancers started, and in the treatments they had received before. The test was "double blind": neither the patients nor the doctors knew who was getting vitamin C and who was getting the placebo. At the end of the study, the researchers found that "the two groups showed no appreciable difference in changes in symptoms, performance, appetite or weight."

There were, to be sure, some curious results. In the course of the study, twenty-seven patients dropped out of the experiment and received neither the placebo nor the vitamin C. When the researchers analyzed all their data, they found that the average survival rate for the 127 patients who received either the placebo or the vitamin C was fifty-one days. But the survival rate for those who had dropped out was only twenty-five days. Perhaps even more puzzling, one patient in particular responded spectacularly well, a man who had been severely ill and who had not responded to any form of chemotherapy. While all the other patients had survived for an average of seven weeks after entering the study, he was still alive more than a year later. And for reasons no one could explain, he had been one of the patients who had been receiving the placebo.

The Mayo Clinic study, however, soon became a source of controversy itself, mainly because Pauling objected strenuously to the way it had been conducted. He had written the Mayo group, Pauling said in a letter to the *New England Journal of Medicine,* and had stressed to them that they "should be careful to use only patients who had not received chemotherapy." In fact, he wrote, Dr. Charles Moertel, one of the principal investigators, had assured him that vitamin C would be tried only in patients who had not been subjected to chemotherapy. Pauling's point was simple enough: The value of vitamin C is that theoretically it helps the immune system battle cancer cells; thus, because chemotherapy severly damages the immune system, vitamin C would be of no value to anyone who had undergone chemotherapy first.

Moertel, Dr. Edward Creagan, another principal researcher, and the other participants in the study had tried to anticipate these objections. In the paper they submitted to the *Journal* they noted that "although patients with advanced cancer who have previously been treated with irradiation or chemotherapy are indeed immunosuppressed, they are not totally incapable of mounting an immune response. One might expect that vitamin C would exert some restorative influence in patients whose immune apparatus has been compromised by earlier treatment efforts."

Nevertheless, Moertel and Creagan were forced to address the question again by replying to Pauling's objections in a letter to the *Journal.* In the first place, they said in this communication, they had made no commitment to use only patients who had not received chemotherapy. Moreover, they said, they had advanced Pauling a copy of their paper before it had been published. Pauling had pointed out that they had not noted in the paper that the patients they had studied had received chemotherapy. To meet Pauling's objections, they added in the letter, they had submitted an appropriate clarification to the *New England Journal of Medicine.*

"Overshadowing such minor quibbling is the major obligation that both we and Dr. Pauling must assume to cancer patients and the general public," Moertel and Creagan wrote to the *Journal.* "On the basis of claims derived from speculation and nonrandomized studies endorsed by the Pauling name, megadoses of vitamin C are being used by thousands of patients with cancer, and such treatment has been embraced by the metabolic therapy cults. Our randomized double-blind study indicates that for at least one segment of the population of cancer patients, such treatment is of no value."

In the meantime, Cameron weighed in with his own observations about the Mayo efforts. What intrigued him in particular was that twenty-seven of the patients originally scheduled for the study had dropped out and had received neither vitamin C nor the placebo. Yet, even those who had received the placebo, Cameron noted, had lived longer than the dropout patients and had managed to survive as long as the group treated with vitamin C.

What was Cameron's very unique explanation for the phenomenon? "I would suspect very strongly that among those patients dying of cancer who gave informed consent to take part in a study to determine whether vitamin C had any value in advanced cancer, many took the precaution of ensuring that they were not in the control group by simply purchasing vitamin C at the corner drugstore," he wrote the *Journal.* "This is a perfectly understandable human response; it could so easily have been checked by simple blood or urine tests."

The Mayo researchers were not taken with Cameron's theories. The twenty-seven nonparticipants, Creagan and Moertel answered, probably died earlier because they were sicker than those in the study. Nor were Creagan and Moertel particularly thrilled by Cameron's implications that the patients in the placebo group had been skulking about, buying vitamin C behind the backs of the researchers. "One could speculate, with equal justification that many of our patients (and his) simply tired of taking all this medication and chucked it down the drain," Creagan and Moertel wrote.

Moreover, after acidly pointing out that as part of their study they had indeed been analyzing urine samples, Creagan and Moertel felt bound to defend not their scientific honor against Cameron's implications but the honor of those patients who had volunteered to participate in the study and who had stuck with it. "All our patients understood they were dying and beyond any hope of definitive treatment," Creagan and Moertel wrote. "They volunteered to participate in this study with full knowledge that they could be assigned to the placebo group and with the hope that they could contribute knowledge of value to others.

"We do not think that it is naive to trust in the sincerity of their altruism or in the honesty of their replies to our regular inquiries regarding compliance."

Although the study conducted at the Mayo clinic has proven— at least to the satisfaction of most cancer experts—that vitamin C is not the magic anti-cancer bullet, the vitamin's role in cancer has been, and still is, the subject of considerable research and discussion.

Within the last few years as research into food additives and preservatives has deepened, scientists have come to the conclusion that some of these chemicals may in fact be carcinogens, compounds capable of causing cancer. One major group under suspicion is the nitrite salts that are added to meat to give it color, to enhance its flavor, or to prevent contamination by bacteria. Nitrites are also produced in the pickling, brewing, and smoking (of fish and meats) processes used by many food companies. In the human digestive tract, these nitrites combine with naturally occurring biochemicals, the amines and amides, to form nitrosamines and nitrosamides. It is these nitrosamines and nitrosamides that, many scientists believe, can cause cancer.

Vitamin C (as well as vitamin E) some food researchers believe, can interfere with the manufacture of the nitrosamines and nitrosamides. In essence, in the digestive tract, the two vitamins compete with the amines and amides for the attention of the nitrites that come into the body via the food. If the vitamins win the race—if they link up with the nitrites—carcinogens may not be formed.

Thus, two Massachusetts Institute of Technology food scientists, Vernon Young and David P. Richardson, were willing to tell an American Cancer Society and National Cancer Institute Conference on Nutrition in Cancer that they "recognize that, in view of the growing evidence concerning the possible causative interrelationships between nitrosamines and ascorbic acid in the incidence of gastric cancer, a case might be made for recommending a moderate level of ascorbic acid in individuals at high risk. In addition, individuals with high risk of cancers of the lower bowel, for example, such as those with polyposis or ulcerative colitis, may also benefit from a supplement of ascorbic acid."

This, however, was no unqualified blessing. Their conclusions, Young and Richardson added, were "speculative and an optimum supplementation schedule cannot be defined, at this stage, if indeed there is one."

Whether speculative or not, the belief that vitamin C may provide some protection against the development of cancer has also been cited, though cautiously, in other NCI literature. For example, in a booklet named *Backgrounder,* the NCI's Office of Cancer Communications points out that "epidemiological studies suggest that lettuce and other vegetables containing vitamin C may offer specific protection of the upper digestive tract."

Backgrounder cites research that seems to indicate that the people in the northern part of Iran suffer a high rate of cancer of the esophagus because their diets are "very low in fresh fruit and vegetables." Similar nutritional deprivations, the booklet says, "have been implicated for the high incidence of stomach cancer in Colombia and Chile." Finally, the publication points out, Japanese who stay in their homeland are at high risk for developing stomach cancer—while children of Japanese who have emigrated to Hawaii have a much lower rate of stomach cancer. "Some investigators suggest that the Western-style diet, including foods rich in vitamin C, may have contributed to this lower risk."

This distinction—that vitamins within a balanced diet may confer protection against some forms of cancer but that vitamins in megadoses do not cure cancer—is particularly important to remember because nutrition scientists and epidemiologists (the people who study the incidence and distribution of diseases in various population groups) are turning up some preliminary evidence that vitamins other than C may also have potential in the fight against cancer—though not necessarily in megadoses. A number of epidemiologists, for example, have looked at the dietary habits of smokers and have found that the smokers who have a good dietary intake of vitamin A are likely to have a somewhat lower risk of developing lung cancer than smokers whose diets are deficient in vitamin A. Similar links between a diet low in A and cancer of the bladder and larynx have also been noted. In fact, by 1982 the epidemiological evidence had grown so strong that the National Research Council, which had undertaken a study of the scientific information on diet, nutrition, and cancer in behalf of the National Cancer Institute, was willing to go on record as saying "the epidemiological evidence is sufficient to suggest that foods rich in carotenes or vitamin A are associated with a reduced risk of cancer." It is important to note, however, that the same NCI report recommended that vitamin and mineral supplements should not be taken in the hopes that they would provide the needed insurance policy against cancer.

Since the 1950s the National Cancer Institute has been funding research into the role vitamin A could play as an anti-cancer drug. In fact, more than a third of all NCI-supported research in the field of chemotherapy is aimed at finding vitamin-A-related compounds that could have an impact on cancer that has already developed. And, as the 1980s came around, NCI also threw some major weight behind studies that would determine if vitamin A in the diet can act as a mitigating agent against the development of malignancies.

One study, being conducted in Hawaii, is still going on. But the other one, carried out by the Louisiana State University Medical Center in New Orleans, was finished in late 1982. It refined even further the concept that the vitamins could influence the onset of cancer. To carry out their analysis of vitamins and cancer, the LSU researchers compared the amount of vitamin A healthy volunteers were consuming with the amount ingested by patients who had lung cancer but who were still alive and by patients whose lung cancer had proven fatal. The patients who had died of lung cancer, the researchers found, had had the lowest levels of vitamin A and of betacarotene, a compound that is present in leafy green and yellow vegetables and which the body uses to make vitamin A.

By carrying their analyses further, the LSU researchers came up with a surprising result: While the data indicated that the lung cancer patients who were still alive had lower levels of vitamin A and betacarotene in their blood than the healthy volunteers, the facts also showed that the patients had been eating foods that were higher in vitamin A and lower in betacarotene that the people who did not have cancer. The conclusion drawn was that perhaps betacarotene is even more important than vitamin A—that the body needs this important vitamin A precursor to maintain a sufficiently high, protective, level of vitamin A circulating in the body. Without the precursor, even a diet very rich in vitamin A may not be sufficient to elicit enough of a safeguard against cancer.

A more definitive answer to the question may come when Dr. Charles Hennekens of the Harvard Medical School finishes a study designed to determine, among other things, whether betacarotene supplements taken every other day will affect the health of some twenty-seven thousand physicians participating in the study.

If the medical establishment is ready to recognize that, in some instances, vitamins may play a role in preventing the onset of cancer, is the establishment being hypocritical when it derides claims that massive doses of vitamins can actually cure this disease?

Not at all. A substantial number of cancer experts are willing to accept the possibility that vitamins in a balanced diet may confer a benefit to people who may risk contracting cancer if their diets are deficient. Accepting that possibility does not pose a danger to anyone, least of all potential cancer patients.

But accepting blindly the idea that vitamins are magical anti-cancer potions does have its dangers—especially when that idea leads to the indiscriminate recommendation that vitamins should be taken, not as a natural part of the diet, but as supplements in often massive doses. Among other things, while there is evidence that vitamins may prevent cancer, there is also evidence that in some cases vitamins may actually promote cancer.

Though vitamin C is hailed for allegedly prolonging the lives of cancer victims, some evidence shows that its role in cancer may not be solely salutary. Some studies have demonstrated that cancerous growths seemed to show a high predilection for vitamin C—that is, that some tumors seem to deplete the body of what stores of vitamin C it has by drawing the vitamin to their own cells. Guinea pigs, for example, like man, do not manufacture their own vitamin C. Scientists studying cancer in these animals have found that their tumors require vitamin C for growth. And researchers studying tissue samples taken from patients with skin cancer, for example, have found that the skin growths contained more vitamin C than the more normal tissues surrounding the growth. Researchers, furthermore, have found that if they combine the vitamin B_{12} with the chemical cis-platinum, they can extend significantly the lives of rats with leukemia. However, in some instances B_{12} actually seems to make a tumor grow faster. This finding is particularly ironic in light of the fact that back in the late 1950s B_{12} was touted, until the claim was proven false, as a cure for neuroblastoma, a cancer that often afflicts children.

The evidence that vitamins may actually contribute to cancer is not limited to animals. Some of the chemotherapies that have proven successful against human cancers do their job by interfering with a tumor's ability to make use of vitamins. The cells in some human cancers, for example, use folic acid in their genetic machinery to help them reproduce themselves. Methotrexate, a powerful anti-cancer drug, does its work by imitating folic acid and fooling the cancer cells into trying to use it to reproduce—thus effectively aborting the cancer's efforts to spread. Some researchers even believe they will make further progress against several forms of cancer if they can pinpoint other vitamins that contribute substantially to a tumor's ability to grow and if they can develop so-called antagonists that stop the vitamin from contributing to the spread of the disease.

The difference in attitude between cancer researchers willing to countenance the possibility that a healthy dose of vitamins in the diet may be beneficial and the faddists who would have us swallow vitamins by the ton is even more clear-cut: No one will suffer any harm if they add oranges, grapefruits, lettuce, and other vitamin C-rich foods to their diet. But anyone who has cancer and who listens to the sermon that massive doses of vitamins—A, C, or E—will help them avoid the horrors of chemotherapy or radiation may suffer problems brought on by the vitamins themselves.

Thus, though there is no evidence that huge doses of vitamin A will cure cancer, many books and pamphlets circulated by food faddists recommend that cancer patients take tens of thousands of international units of vitamin A a day. But a continued intake of such doses can lead to blindness and damage to the liver and bones.

More than a few cancer patients have suffered terribly as a result of massive vitamin A doses prescribed for them by vitamin faddists. The story of Chuckie Peters, as told by his mother, Paulette, to an Illinois Senate subcommittee on medical fraud, is a tragic case in point.

In early 1978, Chuckie's family received the news that their son, seven years old at the time, was suffering from lymphocystic null-cell leukemia. The family was stunned by the diagnosis. What followed was even worse. The boy was subjected to spinal taps, bone marrow aspirations, biopsies—in short, all the painful, traumatic medical procedures that are the cancer victim's lot. The ordeal, of course, was not over. The medical procedures were followed by chemotherapy and radiation.

Because the boy was suffering so much, his family sought alternative treatments. In time, Paulette Peters told the subcommittee, the family was put in touch with a retired Texas physician who was using vitamin A to help enhance "the immune system of persons taking chemotherapy drugs." A telephone conversation with this physician, Mrs. Peters said, led to the conclusion that Chuckie should take 120,000 or more international units of a vitamin A concoction each day. Other vitamin "experts" sought out by the family also agreed that massive vitamin A doses would speed Chuckie to recovery.

The oncologists who had been treating Chuckie warned the family about the possible dangers of vitamin A. But the vitamin faddists who had taken an interest in the boy's case assured her that this dosage was safe. The family, torn by their love for the boy and the conflicting advice presented them, effected a compromise of sorts. They kept Chuckie under the care of the conventional doctors, but continued giving him the vitamin A. In October 1979, Mrs. Peters told the subcommittee, matters came to a climax:

> On October 19, a year after having started Chuckie on the vitamin A therapy, he started having waves of nausea and much itching of the skin.
>
> On October 23, I was called from his school to come and get him—he was very nauseated along with having a severe headache. He started vomiting repeatedly at home and was unable to hold anything in his stomach. The day after, the headaches continued as well as the starting of wrist and skin pain. The pain progressed, in the days to come, to such a point that he could barely walk. Sensitivity to light increased to where the room had to be darkened. He then started showing signs of muscle spasms in his right arm—it would jerk downward as he tried to feed himself. Each day brought more and more pain; he couldn't walk at all and the touching of his arms and legs brought screams of pain.
>
> At this time I wrote (to one of the doctors who had recommended vitamin A) asking for reassurance about the vitamins and also information as to what was happening to Chuckie. He did assure me the problems Chuckie was experiencing had 'never been noted by him nor did he ever read of them in relation to . . . vitamins.'
>
> After thorough examination and blood tests were done on Chuckie (at the hospital where he had been undergoing conventional treatment) excessive levels of calcium were found in Chuckie's blood—a resulting factor of vitamin A toxicity. He was immediately admitted to the hospital and an IV started to help to flush out the calcium from his system.
>
> A brain scan and body scan were scheduled. The brain scan showed swelling in the cranial areas, and the body scan revealed extra bone growth causing much bone inflammation—the reason for the extreme amount of pain experienced.
>
> The only relief Chuckie had from the pain was through the dispensing of the various pain medications: first Tylenol with codeine. Then Demerol. After a while these had no effect on the pain. As a last resort, the doctors administered methadone, starting at 5 milligrams, alternating with Tylenol with codeine every three hours for twenty-four hours. That eventually did not have the desired effect. Methadone was used alone and increased to 7.5 milligrams, then to ten milligrams. Once again the pain was felt—

the methadone no longer seemed to have any effect.

The doctors were beside themselves, not knowing what they could do to help relieve this terrible pain.

Then, by the grace of God, Chuckie started showing signs of improvement—less pain and his appetite started picking up. Two days later he was released from the hospital [but was] unable to return to school for another two and a half months.

Almost half of this time we carted him around in a wheel-chair. His thinking capabilities and concentration were minimal for a time; his weight loss was almost ten pounds. Our son was a shell of what he was a few months before. The three years on the chemotherapy program never yielded the amount of pain Chuckie experienced during that three and a half months of pain from vitamin A toxicity.

We don't know what the benefits of the vitamin A therapy were—we saw much of the negative side effects which almost cost our son his sight—which almost cost him normal brain functions—which almost cost him his life!"

Chuckie's encounter with vitamin A almost proved to be fatal. Fortunately his parents, despite their flirtation with vitamin quacks, had enough sense to keep him under sound medical care. Many other cancer patients probably have not fared as well. Not necessarily because they died of vitamin toxicity but because they listened to the misleading advice of vitamin faddists and gave up conventional treatment. Many of these people have died without knowing they were victims of charlatans.

The conviction among thousands of Americans that vitamins cure cancer and the determination with which quacks, faddists, and researchers eager for admiration and honor seize upon that conviction is only a small part of the mystique and nonsense surrounding vitamins. In a multitude of ways vitamins hold within their grasp millions of Americans, men and women in eager pursuit of easy answers for complicated medical problems, bothersome personal problems, and even minor nuisances that could just as well be ignored. In their own way, vitamins are at the center of a cult that is as powerful as any religious movement that has swept across the nation.

CHAPTER III

Vitamin E:
Snake Oil for the Heart

The road to London, Ontario, is broad and straight, running
through the vast and virtually unbroken plains of midwestern
Canada. The city itself is so densely packed in the midst of un-
ending horizons that it seems as if its residents have crowded
together as closely as possible to find mutual succor against whatever unknown perils might come rolling in at night out of the flat
fields that surround the city.

On one of the city's narrow streets stands an old gray, weather-
beaten but still stately mansion. Once the setting for a novel *(The
Blue Locket* by Frances Sarah Moore, a local writer), it served as
the headquarters of the Shute Institute, where Dr. Evan Shute
reigned as the world's foremost spokesman for vitamin E until his
death in 1978.

Dr. Leo Lutvak, a researcher who had questioned the over-
zealous use of vitamins, had told me he couldn't get past the front
door of the Institute because he was among those hostile to
vitamin E, and so, when I visited the Institute in the mid-1970s, I
approached it with some apprehension. But the unguarded heavy
oak door opened easily into a warm interior of polished and
lustrous cherry-wood ceilings and parquet floors. Italian marble
fireplaces, stained-glass windows, walls covered with embossed
leather surrounded the nurses and aides who were bustling from
large room to large room, talking with patients, checking appoint-

ment books, and answering the hundreds of telephone calls coming from people seeking advice about vitamin E and its uses.

I was early for my morning appointment with Shute, and since he had not yet come to the Institute to start his day, I wandered about the main floor. One room in back, occasionally given over to local community groups for cultural events, was filled with display cases. Inside one glass case was a copy of *The Blue Locket*. In the others were assorted works by and about the Shutes. (Some were published by the Institute, some published by independent publishers. Many of these books have sold hundreds of thousands of copies.) One in particular drew my attention: *Flaws in the Theory of Evolution* by Dr. Evan Shute. "Progress in the biological sciences is rapidly altering the picture of Nature and its species," an ad for the book told me later. "Among the questions considered in this book are such puzzles as these: Why no life in the lower four-fifths of the earth's crust? . . . Did life begin spontaneously? Why no evolution in bacteria? . . . Undoubtedly micro-evolution occurs. But is evolution of the great groups of plants and animals supported by recent evidence? . . ."

"Mr. Fried?" I turned to see a tall, elderly gentleman approaching me. Dr. Shute was impeccable in a well-tailored, conservative blue suit. A kindly face, grandfatherly demeanor, and white hair did not belie, on first impression, that in his youth this man had been, as a public relations writer for the Institute put it, the Canadian Intercollegiate light-heavyweight boxing champion and a "considerable campus personality."

Evan Shute smiled at me engagingly. "May I show you around?"

He led me slowly back into a large room where a group of patients was already waiting to see the doctors who were practicing at the Institute. As we passed, Dr. Shute confided that he was looking for more doctors to join the staff to help share the heavy patient load. Off to one side stood a display, one of those large light-boxes that illuminates pictures at the push of a button or the flip of a switch. With just a barely noticeable tremor, Dr. Shute flipped on the light, and a morbid display of "before and after" photographs jumped into view: ulcerated and gangrenous legs, feet, and hands, their deep wounds marked by red and black torn issues surrounding gaping holes in which parts of the underlying bone and cartilage could be seen—all of them as they allegedly looked before vitamin E was prescribed in massive doses, and all of them as they allegedly looked after the various patients had been treated with vitamin E. Startled, I looked quickly out of the corner of my eye, wondering if the patients in the room should be exposed to this sort of thing. No one was paying any attention, so I turned back to Shute, who was saying something about these being "marvelous" examples of results elicited with vitamin E at the Institute.

We continued walking through two more floors of the Institute. Dr. Shute walked slowly, talking in a low, sometimes tremulous voice, pointing out, with an infirm, slightly wavering hand, table after table made of hand-carved cherry, one empty consultation room after the other, an old fashioned electrocardiograph machine, the Institute's laboratory. I listened to this old man talking—at this point he was telling me that the pamphlets in a rack quaintly marked "Problems Peculiar to Women" were reprints of chapters from a book that was never published because the local medical society objected to its very strong vitamin E orientation—and I felt somewhat puzzled, somewhat sad, and somehow almost cheated. Heart specialists all over the North American continent were gnashing their teeth because seriously ill people wanted to (and, of course, now in the 1980s still do) believe that vitamin E would cure their heart disease (and mitigate other problems as well) and here the prime mover behind the vitamin's continuing success turned out to be nothing more than the old man before me.

According to *The Summary,* a yearly journal published by the Shute Institute when I visited there, Evan Shute decided way back in 1936 that fetal deaths observed in female rats deprived of vitamin E in their diets were due to a change in the supply of oxygen to the placenta. The report in *The Summary* on Dr. Shute's works deftly links him to pioneering work done with vitamin E and rats at the University of California: "The store of Evan Shute's notable work as a medical investigator harks back to 1922 when Dr. H. M. Evans and Dr. K. S. Bishop . . . discovered vitamin E and its value in preventing miscarriage in pregnant rats . . ." There is no evidence that Shute ever worked with the California researchers. It is also interesting to note that Evans and Bishop did not discover that vitamin E prevents miscarriages in pregnant rats. What Evans and Bishop discovered was that, without a small but important dietary allotment of vitamin E, rats had trouble carrying their young to full gestation. The difference is subtle but important.

Following the belief that the miscarriages were due to a changed oxygen supply, *The Summary* says, Shute then had the "hunch" that if vitamin E could play a part in preventing the degeneration of oxygen supply to the rat placenta, it could do the same for human hearts. This quantum leap in medical logic was tested immediately. "A penniless old man, a fellow churchman, was a sufferer from severe angina," *The Summary* recounts. "He had experienced a coronary attack the previous November. Dr. Shute gave him wheat germ oil, the richest source of vitamin E at that time, and the old man gulped it down in large amounts. The result was a tremendous surprise and a vindication of his new theory. The patient's excruciating pain was relieved almost at once; the throbbing in his temples eased entirely; his ears stopped buzzing; he was able to do some gardening; every day he showed improvement."

According to *The Summary*'s official history, Evan's brother, Wilfrid, who had been interning in Toronto, wanted to see for himself whether or not his brother's idea had any merit. Wilfrid gave wheat-germ oil to four cardiac patients in the hospital where he was serving his internship. "What followed was one of the bitter set-backs all research men know, the accident which often causes them to abandon an idea completely," *The Summary* recounts. "The experiment . . . was a total misfire; nothing happened; no patient improved. The brothers decided that the reaction of the old man was a pure fluke. Nothing further was done and the heart secret folded its wings."

But, says the journal in this paean to Shute, the idea that vitamin E could help heart-disease patients was not to be driven from the doctor's head. "The belief that vitamin E had some mysterious connection with the blood vessels, the blood and even the heart had remained hidden in a pigeon hole far back in Evan Shute's mind," the journal says. "It bobbed up now and then to pester him, knocking at the door of his thoughts."

Finally in the mid-1940s, Shute found another chance to pursue his theory that vitamin E could cure problems associated with the circulatory system. Shute asked a senior medical student to run an experiment to determine if a female sex hormone had anything to do with the clotting of blood. The student, a young man named Floyd Skelton, injected dogs with the hormone, and soon the dogs developed hemorrhages (called platelet-poor purpuras) under the skin. Shute then suggested Skelton administer E to the dogs, on the theory that the vitamin would offset the hormonal activity that was causing the hemorrhages. "This was the historic turning point," *The Summary* says. "The dose of vitamin E that Skelton gave the dogs was two to four times the amount Dr. Shute had ever tried on patients. The dog's purpura not only disappeared completely, but a secret came to the surface—the size of the vitamin dose! It was huge in the light of all previous studies."

Having established that the vitamin had a good effect on dogs, Shute began looking around for a human patient suffering from purpura on whom to try the vitamin E in massive doses. Dr. Shute called Dr. Arthur Vogelsang, a London, Ontario, physician who specializes in heart-disease cases, and asked him if he had a purpuric patient at the moment. Vogelsang just happened to have such a patient and agreed to give him large doses of vitamin E. "The reaction was clear," *The Summary* recounts. "The man's purpura responded so dramatically that the blotches of discolouration [*sic*] under his skin vanished quickly and almost entirely. Not only that, but Shute's old slumbering belief was confirmed that vitamin E had power to help heart disease. Indeed, the patient's heart responded to an even more remarkable degree than the purpura. In nine days the man who had been facing certain death in the opinion of his doctors was out of bed and bustling about, helping the nurses with their trays.

"Evan Shute was now sure that he really had something of tremendous importance—a new therapy for sick hearts. Two more severe anginas responded remarkably, one of them his own mother. . . ."

Incidentally, not everyone connected with the rise of vitamin E as a treatment for heart disease has this rosy picture of the vitamin's early days. After the first few papers about vitamin E were published by Shute, Skelton, and Vogelsang, Vogelsang's name disappeared from subsequent publications. Wondering why, I called Dr. Vogelsang and drove out from Detroit to see him on a cold, rainy Wednesday in late November.

Dr. Vogelsang's offices are in a cottage on the other side of London, on an old residential street. It is the traditional midweek Sabbath for doctors, so Dr. Vogelsang leads me through a deserted waiting room and front office to the room where he talks with his patients. The front rooms are all dark, and in the gloom there is an inescapable sense of poverty, a sense that if the lights were to be flicked on, the chairs would prove to be threadbare, scuffed beyond repair. Dr. Vogelsang's own office is very small; a gray venetian blind is drawn closed, hiding the window bearing the lashings of the driving rain. The office is dark too, except for a single light over Dr. Vogelsang's desk. Sometimes as he leans away from the desk, as he delivers a melancholy monologue, the physician disappears into the shadows, only his short-cropped gray hair or his light-blue shirt visible. Somewhere in the outer offices the FM radio, tuned to a local station, plays a classical dirge.

"Shute called me and asked if I had a case of purpura," Vogelsang says, drawing heavily on one of the cigarettes he chain-smokes. "I was copacetic on using tocopherol [vitamin E] because the man was a loser, he would die any day. We put him on 600 international units of E a day. On the fifth day I went into the man's room. He was not in bed, his oxygen had been disconnected. I said why in blazes did no one tell me he had died. The nurse said, died? He's out there helping with the trays."

Vogelsang looks off into the gloom of the office, seeking a vision. He chuckles sardonically. "I have made dillies of mistakes in my life, but telling Shute about the effect of the vitamin on that man's heart was the biggest. I wanted to keep it quiet, but they kept pressing and pressing for a release on the thing. It wasn't ready, but the pressure was on. It hit the local paper as a cure. It hit *Time*.[1] We were deluged. I got ten thousand inquiries from the United States."

Vogelsang stops again. His mood, already low, sinks even further. I am uncomfortable. I don't know if the man is given to open

---

[1] The *Time* article appeared on June 10, 1954: "Out of Canada last week came news of a startling scientific discovery: a treatment for heart disease . . . large concentrated doses of vitamin E. . . . The vitamin helps a failing heart . . . it eliminates anginal pain. It is non-toxic."

emotion, but the barely contained self-pity is edging dangerously close to tears. Vogelsang goes on in his pained, one-tone voice. "Shute was going to be a knight on a white charger, force it down the throats of doctors. My approach was to use it on our patients, and if it worked, fine, and if it did not, that was fine too. But he got the bright idea of getting his brother down here and starting the institute. He was going to become the Lister, the Pasteur of heart disease.

From the day Vogelsang's patient made his "miraculous" recovery, the Shutes were convinced that they had found the answer to heart disease. The institute—funded by loans from their mother and friends (vitamin E manufacturers, some say) and their own money—was launched. *The Summary* was started. The massive effort began to convince the world, doctor and layman alike, that vitamin E would succeed where all other medicines had failed.

The Shutes wrote papers and sought to present their views at medical meetings and symposia. With their active encouragement, two groups were formed—the Vitamin E Society in Canada, the Cardiac Society in the United States—to bring the message of vitamin E directly to the public. The two societies organized scores of public meetings at which the Shutes lectured (as did other vitamin E enthusiasts). The two societies also published newsletters, largely to report the views of the Shutes. According to Carl Muir, a Detroiter who served as an officer of the Cardiac Society and who later left the group to sell vitamin E for a living, the societies were also organized to help members (who totaled more than fourteen thousand at one point) buy vitamin E directly from pharmaceutical houses who agreed to handle the special orders.

By and large, the effort to win the hearts and minds of the medical profession failed as medical researchers around the world rose to oppose the Shutes and their miracle vitamin. (It should be pointed out that scientists don't pick only on "outsiders" like the Shutes. They also delight in trying to prove each other wrong at every opportunity. Often they try because they honestly believe that in science, as in law, only an adversary form of debate will succeed in bringing out the truth. Sometimes they do it because, just like plain, ordinary folk, they are jealous if someone else comes up with a seemingly better idea. "Scientists are emotional people," Dr.

Kaufman of the National Institutes of Health says. "I was working with a famous scientist, trying to reproduce something discovered by another man, something my boss did not believe. At first I came out and said, I guess you are right, my data show that so-and-so is completely wrong. Oh, he was in seventh heaven. A few more experiments later it turned around the other way. I went to my boss and said, I went into more detail, and it looks like so-and-so is right. He made me drop the project right there. He wouldn't let me go on. He was only interested in proving this guy wrong.")

Thus, within four or five years after the first claims for vitamin E were reported by *Time* (and published for medical researchers in the science magazine *Nature*), a number of research teams published papers claiming that the Shutes were wrong, that independent tests of vitamin E proved it to be utterly useless in combating heart disease. The negative studies included:

—One carried out by three English doctors who had given twenty-two of their cardiac patients vitamin E and had found that the vitamin did nothing to alleviate the angina pectoris of which the patients had complained.

—Several studies in New York and Philadelphia in which seventy patients were given between 200 and 800 milligrams of vitamin E with no discernible improvement in their conditions—in fact, a few of the patients seemed to get worse.

—A study at Duke University in which twenty-one patients were given vitamin E and a placebo on alternate months. The patients did not know they were getting placebos. Nevertheless, during the month one patient was receiving the placebo he reported that he was feeling less nervous than he ever had before. Another patient on the placebo swore that the "medicine" had enabled him to lose thirty pounds he had been trying to shed unsuccessfully. In any case, at the end of nearly two years, the Duke researchers reported that vitamin E had conferred "no appreciable benefits . . . there was no significant improvement in symptomatology . . . there was no lowering of blood pressure, no decrease in heart size,[2] no improvement in the electrocardiogram. The changes which were recorded . . . were no more than one might expect in the natural

---

[2] Decrease in heart size would be an indication that the heart was no longer being forced to work too hard.

evolution of their cardiovascular disease.''

The early negative reports from researchers not associated with the Shutes created nearly insurmountable blockades to their efforts to have their vitamin accepted as a viable treatment for heart disease. After that initial spate of negative studies, the Shutes were either barred from, not invited to, or snubbed at medical meetings where they tried to plead their case for vitamin E. Convinced that vitamin E represented another effort to foist a worthless cure on an unsuspecting public, physicians even tried to bar open discussions of the vitamin. When a Montreal businessman, a man who had been treated with vitamin E at the Shute Institute, suggested to his Rotary Club in Montreal that one of the Shutes be invited to speak, the committee in charge of issuing such invitations refused. When another committee eventually came to power, it agreed to extend the invitation—in the process raising a storm of protest by doctors who were members of the Rotary Club. The invitation was finally extended, but not before a compromise agreement had been worked out: the talk on vitamin E would be allowed, but the club would not follow tradition and sponsor the usual radio broadcast of a speech by a guest member. The very thought that the public in Montreal might be convinced of vitamin E's alleged anti-heart-disease powers so terrified the doctors that the local newspaper, the *Montreal Star,* suddenly found itself under a great deal of pressure not to carry a report of the scheduled speech at the Rotary Club. The *Star*'s editors, annoyed at the efforts to censor an idea distasteful to one sector of the community, felt compelled to tell their readers in an editorial that ''certain medical men feel so strongly [about the Shutes' ideas] that they are prepared to go to great lengths to prevent public discussion [of vitamin E].''

In time the Cardiac Society in the United States, too, was forced to close up shop. Low-echelon officials of the United States Post Office, alerted to the fact that the medical community considered claims for vitamin E to be fraught with quackery, barred the Cardiac Society from mailing materials on vitamin E. The decision was appealed, but the Post Office stuck by its guns. It would not allow the use of the mails for their presentations attesting to vitamin E's efficacy in ameliorating heart disease. Deprived of the ability to communicate with its members, the society ceased to exist in 1961.

Despite the concerted pressure, the Shutes have managed to reach a public eager for surefire relief from heart disease. In the books the Shutes have published themselves and in books published by independent publishing houses, the Shutes have presented their arguments in behalf of vitamin E directly to the public jury. In *Vitamin E for Ailing and Healthy Hearts,* Dr. Wilfrid Shute cites example after example from among the thirty thousand or so patients the Shute Institute has allegedly treated successfully with vitamin E. Among them:

—A forty-seven-year-old man who came to the Shute Institute because he had suffered a heart attack and was unable to walk more than one block without suffering severe angina pectoris pains. After five weeks of treatment with alpha-tocopherol, Dr. Shute says, the man rejoined his fife-and-drum-type group and "was able to walk at a military pace up and down hills without pain."

—A fifty-six-year-old farmer who was completely incapacitated after suffering a heart attack and who had been depending on his nephew to look after the farm. One day, five weeks after he had started on vitamin E, the farmer thought he might give the nephew a hand. The older man harnessed the team of horses and began to hitch them to a wagon. One of them, a young horse, became frightened and, with the other horse in tow, bolted. "The patient," Dr. Wilfrid Shute wrote, "dug his heels into the ground, see-sawed the reins, and pulled them to a halt just as they reached the gate."

—A woman who had suffered a heart attack in March, 1953, when she was fifty-six years old and who had been unable to teach for almost ten months after her illness. After two months on vitamin E, Dr. Shute recounted, she was able to resume her teaching duties. "Now aged seventy-one," he added, "she lives normally, has a large vegetable garden, which she tends by herself, and walks daily to the post office and back, a distance of a half a mile without any trouble." [3]

Dr. Shute and other doctors who use vitamin E believe that other physicians who question the validity of the vitamin E therapy

---

[3] This book, one of the major publishing efforts in behalf of vitamin E, was issued with Wilfrid's name as author. On the book's back cover, Wilfrid is represented as the "chief cardiologist" of the Shute Institute. One suspects there might have been some skittishness somewhere about presenting Evan, the first and prime believer in E, but also a gynecologist by training, as the author of the book. But according to

are unable to confirm its value because they are simply not using the vitamin right—either because they don't know much about it or because they are simply closing their minds to it and don't want to take the trouble to carry out proper experiments.

According to Dr. Vogelsang, who has gone on using vitamin E despite his falling out with the Shutes, many people do not benefit from vitamin E because they are taking other preparations that negate alpha-tocopherol's effect. Iron, sometimes given as a supplemental mineral, Dr. Vogelsang points out, is a direct antagonist to vitamin E and will wipe it out completely. Laxatives, Vogelsang says, contain mineral oil and tend to coat the gastrointestinal tract. Since vitamin E is oil-soluble, the medication is absorbed by the oil, not the intestinal tract, and is washed out in the next bowel movement. More important, says Dr. Vogelsang, the soft capsules in which most doctors give vitamin E (including doctors in the United States and, Dr. Vogelsang adds, Dr. Shute) dissolve in the stomach. The stomach's high acid content, Dr. Vogelsang says, destroys one half to two thirds of the alpha-tocopherol before it can be assimilated in the body. Thus, while a patient might require 1,600 international units of vitamin E, he is, if he is taking the soft gelatin capsules, getting an effective dosage of only 800 international units, maybe even less. "I use a product with an enteric coating that goes through the stomach like a marble but opens in the intestine, which is alkaline, and where all of the vitamin E is absorbed," Vogelsang told me. "Shute tried to make a capsule with an enteric covering, but his supplier made it too thick and so the whole thing was excreted. So Shute came out with all these massive doses and the hell with what was destroyed."

There is absolutely no doubt in his mind that vitamin E helps cardiac-disease patients, Vogelsang says. "I took fifteen hundred patients who had had a first infarction and to whom I gave my vitamin E capsules," he says. "Then I hired a statistician who found that only one thirty-seventh of them had suffered

---

The Summary, Evan Shute has come to terms with the dilemma. Talking about Evan Shute's perseverance in behalf of E, *The Summary* notes that Evan Shute's "equable temper" is "not ruffled by the short-sighted comment of cardiologists speaking without trying the therapy. 'What can a gynaecologist know about the heart?' An analogous thing was said about Banting: 'What can a bone surgeon know about diabetes?' " Poor Banting—a man for all comparisons.

recurrences. One the other hand, I have had several recurrences among patients who have discontinued the E or have switched to gelatin capsules. I didn't publish the results, though, because no one would have possibly believed it."

Conventional cardiologists and heart specialists, Evan Shute maintained when I talked with him in his office, were more intent on proving him wrong than in giving the vitamin therapy a fair trial. Moreover, Shute said, once they talked themselves into believing that E does not work, they had painted themselves into a tight corner from which there was no escape.

"They didn't say it was partly wrong," Dr. Shute said angrily and with a good deal of hurt in his voice. "They said it was totally wrong. They condemned everything we had done. Now, even placebos work 40 percent of the time when people have pain, so at least we should have done as well as the placebos. But they had to prove they were right, and so they produced paper after paper, evidence after evidence, that we were totally wrong. It got to the state where they had to be right. If they were wrong, just think of the situation they have gotten into. If we have done such a good thing and they have ignored it for twenty-five years or more, they have tremendous offense to answer for and people will make them pay for it."

Many vitamin E enthusiasts are convinced that the medical profession has been so intent on proving the Shute theory wrong that it has not even bothered to follow the Shutes' basic instructions on how to use the vitamin. In fact, Evan Shute complained in a letter to the *Canadian Medical Association Journal* that "we have been insisting . . . by every means open to us that one should use enough alpha-tocopherol (the scientific name for E) or one is not using it at all; it is comparable to using inadequate doses of insulin in treating diabetes. Surely we have the right to expect that others following in our steps in treating cardiovascular disease with vitamin E should take some cognizance of our suggestions as to dosage."

It is, however, very difficult to sympathize with Evan Shute's complaints that other medical researchers have been unable to duplicate his successes with vitamin E because the doubters did not use the vitamin long enough or in sufficient doses. While the studies that followed the first publications touting the value of E were not perfect in every way, they were based on vitamin E dosages that ranged from 300 to 800 international units of E a day.

It is true that in some instances literature penned by one of the Shutes talks of doses that sometimes range into the thousands of international units of vitamin E. But consider. One of Dr. Wilfrid Shute's early testimonials to vitamin E therapy was a fifteen-year-old boy who was brought under his care because he was in the throes of a second attack of rheumatic fever. "The only treatment I used for the boy was 200 units of alpha-tocopherol daily," Dr. Shute reported. "In three days he was apparently well, and on the sixth day he walked into my office. He was able to return to normal farm activities. . . ." In his *Vitamin E for Ailing and Healthy Hearts,* Dr. Wilfrid Shute cites a forty-seven-year-old woman who reacted well to 375 international units of E, and a forty-one-year-old man who was started on 400 international units of E a day and who "ten days later . . . felt definite improvement, and recovery was nearly complete between the third and fourth week of treatment." It is hard to castigate any research team that, after reading some of the early claims made for E, gave patients 400 to 800 international units of vitamin E for a month in order to test the claims being made by the Shutes.

If medicine has made any progress against disease in the last two hundred years or so, it often has been because researchers have been willing to follow rigorous scientific procedures to test theories of disease and to ascertain the value of new drugs or other medical procedures. We often hear of significant fluke discoveries, the gee-whiz kind of events that tinge medicine and science with an air of romance and mystery. But if Fleming (to cite one of the gosh-dad discoveries), after finding that one of the molds in his laboratory dishes seemed to kill bacteria, had rushed out of his laboratory screaming at all of us to for God's sake eat green mold if we wanted to protect ourselves against infectious diseases, the science of antibiotics (and indeed the world) would not be in very good shape today. It is very conceivable that, without some assiduous followup work on Fleming's part, no one would have taken green mold very seriously and penicillin might have died a-bornin'.

Rigorous studies mean, again, double-blind, strictly controlled experiments. But, like most vitamin enthusiasts, Shute was disdainful of the double-blind study. "Double-blind studies," Shute said to me, "are unethical and immoral. The most outstanding example of a controlled study was that of the diphtheria anti-toxin. When the man who developed the anti-toxin was told to take a diphtheria ward in a hospital in Paris where he worked and treat one-half of the ward and not treat the other half and to see what the controlled studies showed, he refused to do this. It was done by others, of course, and the anti-toxin saved all the children on one side, and a high percentage of the children on the other side died. That was real controlled study and it proved the value of the diphtheria anti-toxin. But wasn't it horrible? It cost a lot of lives.

"You can observe the patient as his own control. You have a patient with a degenerative disease, cardiovascular disease that always goes downhill. You have a patient here at this place on the slope, then this place on the slope, he is deteriorating, always deteriorating. Suddenly you give him a substance and he goes back and runs around like a wild man, he's well again, he goes back to his job. I would say that it was the substance that was responsible."

Shute decidedly was angry. His office in the corner of the Institute's third floor was spacious, warmly lit by a late-afternoon sun. As if posing for a daguerreotype, Dr. Shute sat at this large roll-top desk, which he had opened for work. In talking with me, he grew defiant as he discussed double-blind studies, as he remembered the indignities he had suffered at the hands of established medicine, as he recalled the meetings from which he had been barred, the meetings to which he had never been invited, the meetings where he was not able to set up his display of the miraculous vitamin E cures. He stopped talking for a moment to let the passions cool. But the next thought that crossed his mind set him off again. "There have been no controls on thousands and thousands of people who have had bypass operations. Only the Shutes need controls. Other people who are in cardiovascular work don't!"

The rush of Shute's words carry a certain logic that on closer scrutiny is simply an illusion. Patients, contrary to Shute's assertions, cannot be their "own controls" especially if they suffer from chronic diseases—that is, diseases that take their toll over very long periods of time. If you were to draw a graph of the course a chronic disease takes in a patient, the graph would not show a line plunging straight down. Rather, it would look like a staircase: a brief vertical line, representing a deterioration in condition, a brief horizontal line, representing a stabilization, another brief line down, another horizontal one, and so on.

The "step" course of most chronic diseases (like heart disease, for example) is the reason that people who suffer from chronic ailments are susceptible to quackery. "If they get a [questionable] compound at or near a point where they would level off anyway then the leveling off is attributed to the compound," says Dr. Jess Thoene of the University of Michigan. In other words, rather than attribute the temporary relief from suffering to the natural course of things, the patient who has been desperately seeking a cure attributes his new-found well-being to the magical potion he has discovered. To be fair, the same phenomenon fools the "expert" who has prescribed the potion. "If you have done something at the point [where the patient would have been in a stable period] you think you've done something. But if you follow the patient for [an additional period of time] you would see that you didn't do anything," Thoene adds. The problem, of course, is that in most cases the people who prescribe vitamins for assorted chronic conditions do not keep their patients under long-term observation.

Shute's implication that the coronary bypass operation gained widespread acceptance without scrutiny was also self-serving. As late as the mid-1970s, many heart disease experts expressed grave doubts about the operation's efficacy and in fact often counseled against it. Only recently, as statistics have confirmed that a bypass operation is an effective way of controlling angina pectoris pain, has most of the opposition to the operation diminished.

Moreover, Shute was wrong in implying that members of the medical establishment can impose questionable procedures on the public without challenge. Even surgical techniques have been subjected to double-blind studies. At one point in the history of cardiovascular disease treatments, some surgeons were arguing that the supply of blood to the heart muscle of patients suffering from angina pectoris could be increased by cutting or tying off one of the mammary arteries feeding blood to the chest wall muscles. With one of those arteries cut or tied off, the proponents of the procedure argued, pressures would form above the ligation and would reverberate back along the arterial system until they forced more blood to be diverted into the arteries feeding the heart.

The notion had appeal. And there was one additional advantage to accepting it: Other major heart surgeries required opening the chest wall, stopping the heart, handling the heart. The mammary ligation operation required merely that the surgeon do a skin incision (requiring only a light anesthetic) to reach the mammary artery. Surgeons began performing the operation and soon there was a flood of reports to journals, citing patient after patient cured by the mammary ligation operation and enthusiastically recommending the procedure.

Skeptics, of course, abounded. And finally a group of heart surgeons decided to try a controlled experiment to test the new, highly touted surgery. Patients who were suffering from angina pains and who had sought the operation for relief were admitted into a special surgical program. All of them were properly prepared for the operation and wheeled ceremoniously into the operating room (not at one time, of course). But once they were in the operating room, only half of the patients were actually given the mammary ligation. The other patients were only nicked along the skin—that is, the surgeons opened the skin and stitched it up without touching the mammary artery. After the operations, all the patients (all of whom thought they had gotten the real surgical procedure) were followed by cardiologists (who did not know who had received the operation and who hadn't). Almost without exception, both the patients who had the mammary ligation and those who had not reported that the anginal pain had been considerably reduced. Some of the patients who had had the "sham" operation even reported that their tolerance for exercise had increased dramatically after the operation.

When reports of the "sham" study hit the journals, critics of the mammary ligations laughed themselves silly, its proponents red-facedly slunk away, and the operation was never heard from again.

The experience with the mammary-ligation operation points up another (though familiar) problem: that many agents—be they drugs or surgeries—can have a dramatic effect on angina because angina pectoris is a condition that also has a large psychogenic overlay. That is not to say that angina does not have roots in reality. It does. Angina is brought on by a decreased blood supply to the heart muscle—angina is, in effect, the heart muscle's way of screaming that it needs more oxygen. And, in many patients, the angina is debilitating, it sets in with even the slightest exertion because the blood supply to the heart muscle is so severely curtailed by atherosclerotic deposits in the coronary arteries. However, in a good many people, the extent of the angina is often more a function of the mind than of the blood supply to the heart. There isn't a cardiologist or a heart surgeon in the country who cannot go through his files and pick out a substantial number of "cardiac cripples," people who think they have had heart attacks but haven't, people who have had heart attacks but who report angina pectoris pains out of all proportion to the intensity of indicated damage to the heart or to the amount of blockage present in the coronary arteries—in other words, people to whom angina has become an important (if perverse) factor in their lives.

In fact, it is not just the pain that is important. So is the search for relief—especially if the search stands a chance of yielding a bonus, the discovery of a treatment that is new, that is different. The behavior of these cardiac cripples is the same whether the new treatment is coronary bypass surgery or vitamin E. They all go from center to center, from physician to physician, looking for the magic cure. One can understand the psychology involved: if your pain is special, it merits special treatment, special attention by a sage physician with bold new ideas. All of this makes you a very special person who could recover only under special circumstances. "There is a large psychological component involved in angina," says Dr. T. J. Anderson, head of the department of health care and epidemiology at the University of British Columbia. "And if the doctor thinks he has something magical, if he exudes confidence, the patient senses it. There is no doubt you have to separate the chemical from the psychological effects." Because angina is so markedly affected by psychology and by faith, says Dr. H. J. Kayden of New York University, there has been no dearth of "this-is-it" cures for angina, cures that eventually fade away as their placebo effect wears off. "A disorder that is so relentless and for which medicine has no cure is subject to all sorts of claims," Dr. Kayden says. "People are desperate for an agent to relieve it. I couldn't begin to tell you of the number of agents that over the last fifty years were thought to be helpful and then were found to be of no value. I can imagine a cemetery full of buried drugs and on each tomb I can read the names of illustrious physicians who thought that these were the drugs that would relieve angina."

When we consider any new treatment method—whether it is touted by high-ranking and respected members of the American Medical Association or by a vitamin enthusiast—there is something else that must be taken into consideration. In every disease, including one that involves deterioration of a bodily process, there is always the very real possibility that the disease has stabilized by itself. It is true that many people die in the throes of their first heart attack, that many go on to suffer second, third, fourth heart attacks. But many do not. Many people suffer one heart attack and then, under proper medical management, and with the help of judicious living, live out perfectly normal life-spans.

Thus we have to wonder: if, by virtue of his reputation a doctor draws hundreds if not thousands of patients who have authored for themselves an inaccurate history of angina pectoris pain, if mixed in with these people there are a good number of people who might not have suffered another heart attack under any circumstances, if this is the population on which he bases his belief in vitamin E, can anyone take his recommendations seriously?

Shute argues that double-blind studies are immoral because no physician who has an agent he considers effective can morally withhold it from one half of his patients, just to prove that the other half fared better as a result of its administration. There are two bits of specious thinking involved here. Implicit in Shute's argument is the premise that, without the new agent, half of the patients will die. This is obvious nonsense. In a double-blind experiment involving heart disease, those patients not receiving vitamin E can still be treated with conventional medicines, medicines that, after all, have managed to keep a good many people alive, fairly well, and functioning. People could be kept (as they were in the Anderson study) on nitroglycerin or digitalis while the researchers sought to establish whether or not vitamin E confers advantages above and beyond those conferred by conventional treatment methods. Furthermore, isn't the physician or the researcher who refuses to undertake studies to convince the medical community at large of the effectiveness of his discovery being far more immoral by not conducting those studies before unleashing the "cure" on the world at large? As long as he alone (or in alliance with only a few sympathizers) believes in his regimen, only his patients, perhaps a few thousand, will reap the benefits of the treatment. Hundreds of persons, perhaps millions, who are under the care of skeptical physicians will not. "A double-blind experiment may be immoral," Dr. Anderson says, "but to fail to demonstrate that something may be useful is equally immoral."

In the case of vitamin E, precise experiments to determine its value are very necessary because the theoretical underpinnings for its use are also on shaky ground. Much is made of the fact that vitamin E deficiency leads to cardiac problems in animals. But what is conveniently overlooked is that the evidence is far from consistent. Some animals do develop cardiac disease. But others—including monkeys, man's closest relatives on the evolutionary scale and animals that serve as a testing ground for many drugs before they are tried on people—do not. "The diseases caused by a deficiency of vitamin E vary from animal to animal and involve a variety of systems in different species," says Dr. Robert E. Olson, professor of Biochemistry and Medicine at Saint Louis University School of Medicine. "Skeletal muscle dystrophy is noted in a number of species, but only in certain species is this accompanied by cardiomyopathy. In ruminants, the cardiac disease is severe, in rabbits mild, and in primates nonexistent." And even the fact that *some* animals do develop heart problems is not sufficient reason to prescribe vitamin E for humans, because physiological processes differ radically from species to species. Experiments done on animals give preliminary, seldom definitive, indications of what can be expected in human beings. "If you were a turkey," Dr. Kayden says, "you wouldn't want to be treated with something on the basis of its effect on man."

In his book Dr. Wilfrid Shute argues that there is solid evidence that vitamin E is inextricably linked to heart disease. "It is irrefutable," Dr. Shute writes, "that when new and more efficient milling methods were introduced into the manufacture of wheat flour, those methods permitting for the first time the complete stripping away of the highly perishable wheat germ, the diet of Western man lost its only significant source of vitamin E. Flour milling underwent this great change around the turn of the century, and it became general around 1910. The amount of vitamin E in the diet was greatly reduced, and with the loss of this natural anti-thrombin coronary thrombosis appeared on the scene.'' Before 1910, Shute wrote, death from heart disease was virtually unknown in North America.

While Dr. Shute's argument (actually he is not the only vitamin E enthusiast to suggest it) carries an air of authority, evidence for it is far from unequivocal. In the first place, it can be argued that Dr. Shute probably attaches much too much importance to the role of thrombosis, the formation of clots, in heart attacks. It is true that for a long time medical men thought that most, if not all, heart attacks could be traced directly to the appearance of clots in the arteries leading to the heart. These clots, it was thought, closed off the arteries and brought on heart attacks. And, in fact, anticoagulants, drugs that theoretically keep clots from forming, were developed and prescribed for patients in the hope of preventing repeat attacks. However, in time heart-disease researchers decided that blood clots were not the only villains in the drama and were perhaps not even the most important villains in heart disease. Maybe some heart attacks were caused by heart clots, they decided. But in many patients a more likely explanation, they came to understand, is that most heart attacks are brought on because the heart tissue is denied oxygen by plaques that form on the walls of the coronary arteries, plaques that restrict the flow of fresh blood to the heart muscle, plaques that *sometimes* imprison a traveling clot that shuts off all blood supply to the heart. Moreover, studies with populations that have low vitamin E levels also fail to bear out a consistent correlation between a deficiency in E and an increase in heart disease. In many countries where there is a low vitamin E intake, nutritionists say, there is also very low heart-disease rate. ''In the small group of patients with genetic disorders who have problems absorbing and transporting vitamin E,'' Dr. Kayden says, ''you cannot distinguish an increased rate of heart disease. Although most of these patients are in their teens, several are older and they have not developed ischemic heart disease.''

Vitamin E enthusiasts point to the new milling processes introduced in the early 1900s and the alleged absence of heart disease before that time as proof that E is an important anti-heart-disease agent. They could just as well have studied population patterns and decided that country living prevents heart disease. Before 1910 the population of the United States (as, indeed, of many Western countries where heart disease was to reach epidemic proportions by the 1960s) was overwhelmingly rural. Today, close to 75 percent of the American people live in cities. One could just as well surmise that the lack of exercise (for which there were ample opportunities on the farm) in the city and the excessive stresses of urban life (stresses that were nonexistent out among the waving wheat and the scampering chickens) have been responsible for the increase in heart disease. Or one might just as well look at cigarette smoking—another sizable risk factor in heart disease—and the monstrous increase in cigarette consumption since the turn of the century and conclude that it is the prime and only culprit in the development of heart disease.

Contrary to belief (a belief fervently espoused by vitamin E enthusiasts), it is not exactly accurate to suggest that there was little or no heart disease before 1910. A good many medical historians believe that a substantial number of heart attacks may have been passed off as gastrointestinal distress by unsophisticated doctors. A heart attack is not always a pure and simple thing to diagnose. Even today, when a man suffers pains in the chest or in the abdominal area, many tests, including a highly technical and sophisticated search for CPK enzymes, enzymes present in muscle tissue and released by heart tissue in large amounts during a heart attack, are often necessary before a final diagnosis is rendered. One reason for all the tests is that part of the nervous system that services the heart services also other areas near the organ, including the jaw and the gastrointestinal tract: thus, the many men who wake up in the middle of the night believing they are suffering a severe attack of indigestion that later turns out to have been a full-blown heart attack. One more point here: many cardiologists today believe that there is ample opportunity, if sophisticated tests are not used, for some physicians to *overdiagnose* the presence of heart disease. Not a few patients who come to leading heart-disease institutes after being told by their physicians that they have suffered a "little heart attack'' are ultimately found to be in perfectly good cardiac health. One more reason, in fact, to question whether all those people cured or helped by the Shutes do indeed owe their health to vitamin E.

There is evidence that heart disease and heart attacks did in fact pose health problems of considerable magnitude before the turn of the century, before millers began to refine wheat. According to Dr. Robert E. Hodges, professor of medicine at the University of California at Davis, medical textbooks of the very early 1900s describe quite clearly heart-disease problems in the nineteenth century. One book Dr. Hodges found describes, he says, a disease process ''which in my view was unquestionably coronary heart disease in its many manifestations. Physicians of those days, however, used somewhat different terms, including 'hypertrophy and dilation of the heart,' 'atrophy of the heart,' 'myocarditis,' 'endocarditis,' 'fatty degeneration of the heart,' 'thrombosis of the heart' . . . In fact these authors even described 'myocardial infarction as a result of atheromatous occlusion of the coronary arteries,' and quoted medical papers of the eighteenth century which described the disease. The facts are that coronary disease is not a new condition which suddenly appeared after we began to eat white bread.'' And, according to the *British Heart Journal,* as early as 1819 doctors described heart conditions whose ''clinical features included a languid, feeble circulation, oppression in the chest, distress in breathing, coma, syncope, rupture of the heart and sudden death.''

One doctor in the 1850s, the *Journal* says, described eighty-three cases of illness he associated with the heart. A careful examination of the doctor's records, the *Journal* says, revealed that fifty-two of the eighty-three cases were ''examples of ischaemic (CQ) heart disease and that many of the specimens from cases of sudden death or ruptured heart were examples of acute infarction.''

What, though, can one say about all those pictures of the gangrenous and ulcerated limbs and the claim that vitamin E had been the key factor in saving them from amputation? For starters, it may very well have been possible that the people who came to Shute had not received very good care for their problems before they came to his Institute. Many of Shute's critics, even while scorning his belief in vitamin E, acknowledged that he often dispensed otherwise sound medical advice. Thus, we can assume that the people who hobbled into the Shute Institute probably got some very good medical attention in addition to receiving vitamin E—and that it was that attention, not the vitamin, that was responsible for the miraculous cures of the gangrenous and ulcerated limbs. The same thing, obviously, might be said of the people who came to Shute seeking help for cardiovascular problems like heart disease. While some may have been helped by the placebo effect inherent in the dispensation of vitamin E, others undoubtedly benefited from other very conventional, and very sound, advice given by the Shute Institute doctors.

One question that was persistently bothersome to me as I researched the vitamin E question was why, in the face of strong evidence to the contrary, Shute persisted in believing, almost blindly, in vitamin E. Ultimately the simple answer dawned on me. It was not just that Shute wanted to believe in vitamin E. It was that he really was not able to understand the difference between meaningful and fanciful evidence for the vitamin.

That answer began to form in my mind at a roadside diner on the way home from London. One of the features on the light-box back in the Institute's waiting room had been a set of pictures of a dog's heart. As I sat and dunked a doughnut into my coffee while leafing through a couple of issues of *The Summary* that Dr. Shute had given me, the same two pictures stared out at me. One picture, on the left, showed a portion of the heart muscle with one fairly large artery branching off into three major subsidiary vessels and a few scrawny, smaller vessels. The circulatory system is atrophied because the researchers, it is pointed out in material accompanying the pictures, had tied off the main vessel. The picture on the right showed a portion of heart muscle suffused by fat, healthy arteries and scores, if not hundreds, of tiny additional blood vessels. That new blood vessel network, the reader is informed, was the result of vitamin E. The first implication is that vitamin E has helped this dog sprout a new, mammoth blood-vessel system that helped keep the heart well fueled with blood, after the artery was ligated. The second implication is that anyone taking massive doses of vitamin E would not have to worry about a heart attack that might be brought on if a main artery supplying the heart muscle with blood were to be blocked off by atherosclerosis, because the vitamin E would have helped the heart develop a similar blood-vessel network that would bypass the atherosclerotic obstruction and would keep the heart well supplied with blood.

Cardiologists, particularly those who do research with dogs, know that the canine heart is very adept at developing this sort of auxiliary blood-vessel system (it is called collateral circulation) spontaneously. In the second place, cardiologists generally accept that in some people—for reasons that are not entirely clear—a collateral circulation system expands spontaneously when one or two of the main arteries are blocked by atherosclerosis. When the expansion does occur—and unfortunately it does not happen consistently or often enough—the patient with the expanded system may indeed be spared a fatal heart attack because fresh blood is brought to the area previously served by the blocked vessels. Researchers at the Cleveland Clinic in Cleveland, Ohio, have found that men who have two blocked arteries but who have developed expanded collateral circulation have a heart-attack death rate that is 15 percent lower than men who have two blocked arteries but no expansion in the collateral circulatory system. Is it possible that some people unknowingly take doses of vitamin E sufficient to encourage or stimulate the expansion of collateral circulation? The question is not a valid one, because the doses of vitamin E recommended by the Shutes for heart-disease patients runs into hundreds of international units (in some cases, thousands of international units) of the vitamin, far more than is available in the common diet.

More important, the pictures, actually taken by a Spanish researcher, are probably not what they seem to be. The caption accompanying the pictures in *The Summary* implies the photographs were taken in the same dog. Chances are good to excellent, a UCLA cardiology expert who does full-time research with dogs told me, they were not. Photography of the blood-vessel system in the heart muscle is done today through a process known as angiography. An opaque dye is injected into the blood vessels and an X ray is then taken of the heart. The X rays show where the arteries are and indicate if there is free flow of blood through them and, if not, where the major blockages are in the way of proper circulation. Even today, the process, although highly sophisticated and helpful in diagnosing atherosclerotic heart disease, leaves a good deal to be desired. Angiography cannot help the cardiologist photo-graph the smallest blood vessels in the heart muscle. Yet the pic-tures shown in *The Summary* were taken in 1955, a time when the method was still in its infancy, and they purport to show tiny ves-sels that cardiologists and heart surgeons today would give their eye teeth to be able to see.

How, then, were these pictures taken? The UCLA researcher believes that probably through a process known as corrosive cast-ing. In this process a liquid plasticlike solution is injected into the heart vessels of an experimental animal (presumably just before it is sacrificed). After the plastic hardens, the heart is removed from the by now dead animal and is dipped in acid. The heart muscle is eaten away, leaving behind the plastic, hardened into a perfect rep-lica of the circulatory system within the heart. The pictures in *The Summary* look very much like those taken of a heart after corrosive casting. It is very probable, because the procedure kills the animals involved, that the two pictures are of two different dogs. One did have an impaired circulatory system. One did get vitamin E and did have a massive auxiliary circulatory system. The Shutes believed that the vitamin E supplements fed the second dog had to be responsible for this healthy arterial network. They simply ignored the fact that, as in many dogs, that collateral system had probably been in place before the vitamin was administered. For them, the equation was simple: Dog gets E. Dog is seen to have a superb cardiovascular system. Therefore E is equal to increased blood circulating through the heart. In their defense, it must be said that the crude testing methods available in the mid-1950s probably were partly responsible for aiding and abetting the fallacious thinking the Shutes had engaged in. Nevertheless, knowing this, they might at least have read up on canine physi-ology before using dog experiments to sustain their theory about vitamin E.

(The Summary does more than present "evidence" vitamin E is everything its detractors say it is not. The magazine also pre-sents "evidence" that scientific and medical circles ostracize not only the Shutes but others whose ideas and actions have run counter to established beliefs. A deft way to hint that E and the Shutes are not the only victims of establishment opposition: In the 1971 issue of the journal there is an article abstracted from

Science, the magazine of the American Association for the Advancement of Science, which deals with the award of a Nobel Prize in physics to a Swedish physicist, Hannes Alfven. "For a good deal of Alfven's career, his ideas were dismissed or treated with condescension," *The Summary* quotes from *Science.* "He was often forced to punish his papers in obscure journals . . . It is almost (but not quite) incredible to realize that at no time during his fruitful years was Alfven recognized as a leading innovator by his fellow scientists. . . .")

The 1971 *Summary* finds another man who suffered at the hands of his colleagues: Dr. Edward B. Diethrich. Diethrich is a Phoenix, Arizona, heart surgeon who is one of the nation's leading advocates of coronary bypass surgery. Diethrich, after a long apprenticeship under Dr. Michael DeBakey, the famous Houston, Texas, heart surgeon, came to Phoenix to open his own heart institute. Because Diethrich is young, brash, and not publicity-shy, his presence and efforts in Phoenix thoroughly antagonized the established medical community in that hot desert town.

Some doctors tried to fight Diethrich by spreading rumors that his patients were dying left and right. Others tried to get rid of him by pressuring the hospital where Diethrich operated, and where he opened his institute, to curtail his surgical suite privileges. *The Summary* quotes from a *Life* magazine article about Diethrich. "Many Phoenix doctors, who tend to be conservative and treasure the idea of individual practice," *Life* correspondent Rick Gore wrote, "have reacted to Diethrich's new Institute like a desert rattler that has been stepped on. . . . Diethrich lays much of the local antagonism to jealousy and the fact that his new technology threatens to make obsolete 'the old guys with 40 years expertise reading resting EKG's.' Still their hostility hurts. 'Why,' he asks, 'when what we stand for is right and good, and we are all trying to do just a super job, do they attack us? I guess I live in a glass house. I thought everyone would say Doctor Diethrich and his team are great and do wonderful things. . . .'" I can almost see Dr. Shute standing by the huge window in his office, gazing down at the institute's sprawling front yard, silently shaking his head as he commiserates with Dr. Diethrich's sad lament.)

The powers ascribed to vitamin E do not start and end with heart disease. The vitamin has been put forward as an answer to virtually every serious (and not so serious) human ill. It has been proposed as a cure, ameliorating agent, or powerful aid for well over sixty diseases or conditions, including athletic performance, fertility, impotence and frigidity, lupus erythematosus, myasthenia gravis, amyotrophic lateral sclerosis, muscular dystrophy, kidney disease, peptic ulcers, cancer, constipation, cystic fibrosis, diaper rash, warts, detached retinas, hemophilia, and bursitis, to name a few.

It is essentially self-defeating to try to knock down every claim made for vitamin E. But it is hard to take all of them seriously because a good many of them—if not most—evaporate on closer scrutiny. In many animals, it is true that a severe vitamin E deficiency, induced by feeding them a vitamin-E-free diet, ultimately leads to a muscular degeneration. But the kind of muscular dystrophy that is brought on in mice or rabbits by starving them of vitamin E has nothing to do with the kind of inherited, genetically controlled muscular dystrophy that is prevalent in man.

"Studies of dystrophies induced by vitamin E deficiency in animal models have yielded valuable information about genetic human muscular dystrophy," says Dr. A. L. Tappel, a nutrition expert at the University of California at Davis. "Although they are similar in many elements of biochemical and cellular pathology, the nutritional animal dystrophies and the genetic human dystrophies are quite different." Finally, says the National Research Council, the muscles of a person with muscular dystrophy have very normal amounts of vitamin E in them. A lack of E in the diet, or even a theoretical inability of the body to use E available in the diet, have nothing to do with the human version of the disease.

Vitamin E, it is said, can make it possible for a woman who has had miscarriages to bear children. Women who have had one, two, three, and even more miscarriages, enthusiasts claim, have borne children after they were treated with vitamin E. But some very mundane statistics take the edge off that claim. A woman who has not had vitamin E and has had one miscarriage has an 80 percent chance of bearing a child on her next try. A woman who has had two miscarriages has a 62 percent chance of bearing a healthy child without any kind of medical help. A woman who has had three miscarriages has a 27 percent chance that her next pregnancy will come to fruition. Even a woman who has had four miscarriages—a pretty discouraging situation— has at least a 6 percent chance of ultimately bearing a child. It can be argued that, if a woman who has had one, two, or several miscarriages is given vitamin E and subsequently delivers a child, the vitamin, in all probability, had nothing to do with her successful pregnancy.

To say that all of the wondrous tales spun about the powers of vitamin E are just so much fanciful speculation is not to say that the vitamin is without value, that it plays no discernible role at all in human health.

Vitamin E burst upon the world back in 1923 when two University of California researchers were studying the effects of nutrition and diet on the fecundity of laboratory rats. The rats had been fed meals thought to be fully nutritious at the time and were doing well—or so it seemed. All physiological signs indicated that the rats were healthy and thriving. But when it came time for them to reproduce, something was going wrong. The female rats were getting pregnant, they were carrying fetuses. But many of the fetuses were dying before they were born and were reabsorbed by the mother's body. To find out what, if any, ingredient in the diet might help the rats with their reproductive problems, the researchers began adding other foods to the feed placed in the cages. When they got to wheat germ and lettuce, they hit the jackpot: the females began delivering full-term, healthy little rats. Some new, previously unsuspected nutrient, the researchers proposed, was necessary if rats were to maintain their ability to procreate. In 1936 the specific vitamin, given the letter E for popular identification, was isolated in wheat-germ oil.

In what has to be an example of one of the more improvident baptisms of a new substance in research history, the new vitamin was given the scientific title of tocopherol. "If one wonders why the vitamin is worshipped as the stuff that flows from the fountain of youth, he has only to look at what the Greek words really mean," Dr. Tappel writes. *"Tokos* means childbirth and *-pher* means to bear or bring forth. The *-ol* designates it as oil soluble. Thus *tocopherol,* the oil of fertility."

If Shakespeare had asked in 1937 what's in a name, he would

have gotten a one-word answer where tocopherol was involved: derision. The name "oil of fertility" (or some such variation) cast a pall over the vitamin. Few scientists, it seemed for a while, could even mention the vitamin without chuckling.

But the task facing vitamin E researchers was not complicated just by the fact that someone had chosen an unfortunate name for the substance. As the years went by, vitamin E itself was giving researchers headaches. They were simply unable to pin down a definitive and consistent physiological problem that might be associated with vitamin E deficiency in all animals. Ascorbic acid researchers could point at scurvy as the primary result of vitamin C deficiency in animals. Nicotinic acid researchers had pellagra's defeat to brag about. Other vitamin researchers could point to beriberi, rickets, or xerophthalmia as vitamin-deficiency diseases that inexorably appeared when one or another vitamin was denied to all experimental animals. Vitamin E researchers had no such deficiency disease.

Over the years, of course, vitamin E researchers learned a good deal about the chemical structure of vitamin E—that there were in fact various tocopherols, differing in their chemical composition and some of their biological properties; that one of the main functions of vitamin E is to protect polyunsaturated fatty acids in the body, to guard them, that is, against excessive and promiscuous oxidation. But they learned nothing productive, nothing applicable in very practical terms, about vitamin E's larger role in the physiological process. Different species of animals, put on diets stripped of vitamin E, showed a wide and often bewildering array of illnesses and problems. Rats, it was found, suffer a kind of muscular weakening and find it impossible, after continued E deprivation, to stand up. Autopsies of rats sacrificed after vitamin E deprivation revealed that the livers of the animals deteriorate, that some of the organs undergo discoloration, and that the skinlike covering (the epithelium) of the hundreds of tubules within the kidney degenerates. In some animals, namely, monkeys, dogs, calves, and pigs, vitamin E deficiency brings on a muscular degeneration as well. But not in others. In some animals, vitamin E deficiency leads to a severely damaged circulatory system. Not all animals, but a few, do show discoloration of the teeth when they are starved for E. In some species, but again not all, the respiratory system suffers under

E deprivation. But no single thread ever appeared that would have enabled researchers to tie vitamin E to a specific, across-the-board physiological catastrophe that would produce damage in all animals if the vitamin was withdrawn. Thus no scientist was, for a while, able to tell the public "YOU need vitamin E or else surely the following will happen. . . ."

Because it seemed unlikely that vitamin E had no function at all in human beings—even if vitamin E deficiency or problems attributable to an E deficiency were not readily obvious—and because it also seemed likely that humans do need some basic amount of the vitamin, in 1953 the Food and Nutrition Board of the National Research Council commissioned Dr. M. K. Horwitt and the Biochemical Research Laboratory at Elgin State Hospital in Elgin, Illinois, to try to carry out a definitive study of the impact of vitamin E on human beings.

Because the experiment would have to run for a substantial amount of time, Horwitt "recruited" thirty-eight men who had been committed to the state mental hospital for a long time and who would in all probability live out their days at the institution. He placed nineteen of the men on a diet especially designed to be as free as possible of vitamin E (not an easy task, since there is some tocopherol in almost everything we eat). Nine men were given the same vitamin-E-free diet, but were given the tocopherol in 15-milligram dosages in supplemental capsules. Ten men just went on eating the same hospital food they had always eaten.

As the years went by, the amount of vitamin E levels in the blood of the men who were getting none of the vitamin slowly fell. At the end of two years the vitamin E levels in the nineteen vitamin-E-deprived men were nearly half what they had been at the beginning of the experiment. In time the levels dropped to a very low 20 percent of normal. Yet, despite this drastic drop, after eight years of vitamin E deprivation, continuing checkups and tests showed that the nineteen men were in generally satisfactory health and had, in the time since the experiment had begun, developed no physical (or additional mental) problems. The only physiological change that caused the researchers some concern was a drop in the longevity of the patients' red blood cells. That is, while normal red blood cells live an average of 123 days, the red blood cells in the men on the vitamin-E-poor diet were living only an average of 110 days. And since monkeys that had been fed diets deficient in vitamin E developed severe anemias that were extremely difficult to reverse, Horwitt discontinued the experiment rather than chance irreversible damage to the men. As a result of Dr. Horwitt's work, the National Research Council decided to recommend that adults should have about 25 to 30 international units of vitamin E a day.

The strongest indication that vitamin E fulfills some useful function in man came in the mid-1960s, when a number of doctors and researchers caring for and studying prematurely born infants found that some of these babies were developing hemolytic anemia —an anemic condition in which the red blood cells are destroyed long before they live out their normal 120-day life-span. As they worked to discover why the anemia was striking just some babies, the doctors found that the disease seemed to be confined to children who were being nurtured on a commercially mixed substitute. When the milk product was analyzed, it was found to be low in vitamin E. When blood samples taken from the ill babies were analyzed, they too were found to be abnormally low in alpha-tocopherol. And when the babies were fed supplemental vitamin E, their condition slowly improved. It was obvious, then, that premature babies who were neither breast-fed nor given cow's milk but who were given other commercially synthetized products had to have vitamin E. Taking this into consideration, the Food and Drug Administration ordered that commercial milk substitutes used to feed premature babies had to be fortified with vitamin E. The discovery that vitamin E played a vital role in the development of premature infants brought a sense of relief to scientists who were beginning to despair of ever finding an identifiable role for vitamin E in human health. Even the venerable *New England Journal of Medicine* was moved to editorialize recently on the findings, telling the medical world that "E May Be For Excellence After All. . . ."

Neither the finding that vitamin E helps premature infants ward off hemolytic anemia nor the National Research Council's decision to include vitamin E in its list of nutrients that should be taken by human beings went very far toward relieving the uncomfortable feeling among many scientists that vitamin E was still somehow making fools of them. In 1970 two nutrition experts, Sir Stanley Davidson and Reginald Passmore of the University of Edinburgh, complained that "vitamin E is one of those embarrassing vitamins that have been identified, isolated and then handed to the medical profession with the suggestion that a use should be found for it, without any satisfactory evidence to show that human beings are ever deficient of it or even that it is a necessary nutrient for man." And as late as 1973 Dr. Tappel, who holds two professorships at the University of California,[5] wrote that "there is the nagging suspicion that there is a very important use for the vitamin and we are just not smart enough to see it."

Yet, in relatively quiet fashion, many researchers have been working hard to determine the functions of vitamin E. At Colorado State University, Robert P. Tengerdy and Rollin H. Heinzerling of the school's Department of Microbiology, have found that mice and chicks fed moderately high amounts of vitamin E—three to four times the amount they would get in a normal diet—seem able to resist infections better than animals fed normal amounts of vitamin E. The researchers have found that animals fed the supplemental vitamin E seem to have more of the special cells in the body that manufacture antibodies, the "soldiers" that fight infectious agents. The blood of the animals given supplementary amounts of E also contained more of the antibodies themselves. According to Dr. Tengerdy, test-tube experiments have shown that when vitamin E is mixed with the tissues that manufacture the antibodies, the resultant decrease in oxidation within the tissues creates an environment in which the antibody-manufacturing cells multiply at an increased rate. However, stresses Tengerdy, there is no direct evidence that vitamin E has the same effect in a living organism such as a chick or a mouse (much less a human being). "We are not even sure that the vitamin E is directly responsible for the resistance to infections in the mice or chicks," Tengerdy says. "We don't know whether the increased protection is caused by the E or by a function the E helps along. And, it is too early to tell if E, in similar fashion, would help man with his immunological process."

A number of doctors have also reported success with vitamin E in treating intermittent claudication, a disease in which circulation in the legs is impaired, leading to a sometimes excruciating pain during walking and, in some cases, gangrene and amputa-

---

[5] One in nutrition, one in food science and technology.

tion. Patients with severe intermittent claudication are often able to walk no more than a few feet before the pain, set off by muscles starving for oxygen, sets in.

One of the first reports of vitamin E's alleged ability to alleviate intermittent claudication came from the Manchester Royal Infirmary in England. According to the researchers who conducted the study there, more than fifteen hundred patients with intermittent claudication were treated with vitamin E, and most responded in some positive fashion to their unusual therapy. A typical patient, a man they call J.B., the researchers reported, was treated with 400 international units of vitamin E a day from 1948 to 1955. Throughout the seven years he made what was considered to be remarkable improvement. But in November of 1955 he decided to stop taking his vitamin E. Within one year, the researchers say, his condition deteriorated, and instead of being able to walk nearly half a mile before he began to have pain in his legs, he could barely walk 1,200 feet before having to sit down to rest. When he was put back on vitamin E, his condition improved once more.

To prove to themselves the worthiness of the vitamin E therapy, the English researchers conducted a double-blind study with thirty-three patients suffering from intermittent claudication. The patients were divided into two groups, seventeen patients in one, sixteen in the other. Insofar as possible, the groups were "matched" so that the patients in each had nearly the same characteristics. In both groups there were patients who had suffered from intermittent claudication between 6 months and 5 years. In one group the average duration of the disease had been 24 months, in the other 24.4 months. The average age in one group was 58.8 years, in the other 57.4 years. One group was given vitamin E therapy; the other, conventional treatment. After a little more than three months, the patients in the group receiving alpha-tocopherol found that they could walk nearly two hundred yards farther than before treatment. By comparison, the patients in the other group had increased their walking capacities by only some sixty yards.

In a more recent study of the effect of vitamin E on intermittent claudication, a Swedish surgeon, Dr. Knut Haeger, studied 227 patients with the disease. Haeger gave 104 of the patients 300 to 600 international units of vitamin E a day (nothing else). The remaining patients—123—he treated with other medicines, including drugs to

dilate the blood vessels, drugs to prevent clotting, and even mul-
tivitamin preparations. The patients were followed for various
lengths of time, ranging from two to nine years. The results in the
Vitamin E group were impressive. During the course of the study,
one patient who had been on vitamin E lost his leg to amputation
because the claudication ultimately cut off all blood supplies to the
leg. On the other hand, 11 of the patients treated more conven-
tionally had to undergo amputations. According to Haeger, 75 percent of the patients treated with E increased their walking abilities
by 50 percent. Only 20 percent of the patients treated in other ways
increased their walking capacities by the same amount. Furthermore, 38 percent of the vitamin E patients were able to double their
walking capacities, whereas only 4 percent of the other patients
were able to achieve the same goal under conventional treatment
regimes.

Intermittent claudication is probably the only condition in which
the use of alpha-tocopherol in massive doses finds some acceptance
among some establishment doctors. Even those doctors who are un-
remittingly hostile to the slightest whisper of vitamin E in the same
breath as heart disease give some grudging credence to the claims
that alpha-tocopherol can ameliorate the pain and suffering of intermittent claudication. But even here some skepticism is in order.
One of the most common ways of assessing the effectiveness of *any
drug* in mitigating intermittent claudication during its early stages is
to measure how far the patient can walk before and after he is given
the medication before pain sets in. But again, the perception of pain
in walking is often heavily influenced by the patient's feelings. According to at least one critic of vitamin E, the Swedish studies, far
from being scientifically precise, actually conditioned the patients
to expect some change after they were given vitamin E. The study,
he says, primed them to feel better. "It turns out," the critic, a
leading National Institutes of Health researcher, says, "that they
told the patients not to expect anything for four to six months. So,
naturally, at the end of the four months, the patients started looking
for good results." Others agree that the effect of vitamin E on intermittent claudication might be more psychological than physiological, that the vitamin helps patients believe that they are not
hurting as much as they did before and therefore enables them to
walk somewhat farther before giving in to the pain. "There is an

English professor who was taking three grams of vitamin E a day," Dr. H. J. Kayden of New York University says of a man who was asked to participate in a study of alpha-tocopherol's role in circulatory diseases such as intermittent claudication. "He was asked to stop taking the E, but at the end of sixty-four hours he said he didn't want to participate in the study anymore because the pain was coming back. Ultimately, he needed surgery anyway because he was getting such severe pain. When they performed blood analyses, they found that he had very high levels of E even when the pain was at its worst."

Just as some doctors and researchers have been willing to toy with the idea that E may be effective against intermittent claudication, some have been willing to give increasingly serious consideration to the proposition that vitamin E may serve as a deterrent to fibrocystic breast disease, a condition that affects an estimated 20 percent of American women. While the condition, which manifests itself in small lumpy bumps, is often uncomfortable and sometimes painful, it is harmless. However, cancer specialists believe that the woman who has recurring bouts of fibrocystic disease runs a high risk of developing breast cancer—a risk that is two to eight times greater than the risk faced by women who have never had fibrocystic disease.

In at least one experiment conducted by Dr. Robert London, professor of gynecology and obstetrics at Johns Hopkins University, some fairly high doses of vitamin E seemed to give some women protection against fibrocystic disease. London treated more than two dozen women with a placebo and with 600 international units of vitamin E a day for eight weeks. In ten of the women the lumps shrunk while the women were on the high vitamin E dosages.

It should be noted however, that the results of the experiment did not turn London into a vitamin E enthusiast. While the results of his work were encouraging, he told *Medical World News,* they did not constitute an unqualified endorsement of vitamin E— because researchers did not really know yet how the vitamin acts as it does, because it is, in large doses, a drug, and because according to some preliminary evidence, vitamin E acts differently in different women.

A number of researchers—including scientists at the University of Southern California, the Battelle Institute of Ohio, and the California State Department of Public Health—believe that vitamin E may play an important role in protecting the lungs against damage from air pollution.

According to these researchers, nitrogen dioxide and ozone, the two major components of air pollution—particularly in the photochemical smog that is so prevalent in Southern California—damage the cells in the tissues of the lungs by breaking down several of the cell's component parts, including those that are composed of molecules bearing polyunsaturated fat. Scientists studying lung tissues have also found that the cells do have natural defenses against the pollutants and their destructive effects, and that the most important "protector" seems to be vitamin E. Rats deficient in vitamin E and rats fed diets containing a normal or slightly higher than normal amount of E were exposed to the damaging pollutants. The vitamin-E-deficient rats suffered greater lung damage than those who had normal vitamin E levels.

The research with rats, researchers emphasize, does not mean that everyone exposed to air pollution needs to gulp down vitamin E in massive doses. "It is probable," says Dr. Tappel, one of the researchers who believes that E can protect the lungs against damage, "that the human lung is protected by dietary vitamin E, and it is fortunate that the average U.S. diet supplies a reasonable amount. We should be concerned about people whose diets are low in vitamin E, if those individuals live in cities that have photochemical smog. If these animal experiments have a further message, it would be that probably a level in the range of the RDA [recommended daily allowance], 20 to 30 international units for adults, could be recommended for persons exposed to photochemical smog."

Vitamin E investigators are also fascinated by some tenuous evidence they have found linking the vitamin to some biochemical activities in the body, activities that are responsible for the aging process. Some researchers have found that the appearance in various parts of the body of a pigment called lipofuscin can be correlated with an increase in age and with the level of vitamin E in the body. Lipofuscin apparently cannot be detected in humans under the age of ten but is found in increasing amounts in older people. Specifically, the compound is not present in the heart muscle of youngsters but does occupy as much as 10 percent of the space between the cells of the heart muscle in older people. Theoretically, the pigment accumulates over the years as oxidative processes are carried out in the body. At least one researcher, moreover, has found that lipofuscin seems to accumulate much faster and to a greater degree in the nerve cells of young rats fed a vitamin-E-deficient diet than in older rats fed normal amounts of vitamin E throughout their lives. Other researchers have noted that another pigment—called ceroid pigment—is also found in great amounts in the smooth tissue, skeletal muscle, sex glands, and other tissues of rats fed diets lacking vitamin E.

Ceroid pigment, some researchers feel, accumulates naturally as the organism ages. But, some add, the pigment seems to accumulate faster in the nerve cells of vitamin-E-deficient young rats than in older rats not denied a normal amount of vitamin E. Vitamin E deficiency, some have speculated (though they have not advocated massive vitamin E doses), may contribute to the deposition of ceroid pigments in the nerve cells of man—a deposition that in turn cuts down on the efficient workings of the nerve cells and contributes substantially to the aging process.

For a time, Dr. Tappel was convinced—although, like a good scientist, he changed his mind when further work proved him wrong—that the evidence of vitamin E's role in aging was strong enough to suggest that it might be used prophylactically, not to stave off senility and death forever, or even a substantial amount of time, but enough to put some restraint on the aging process.

That we all, with but a few exceptions, seem to die between the ages of seventy and seventy-five, Dr. Tappel suggested a few years ago, seems to indicate that some outside force—he thought it to be naturally occurring radiation—wages war against our cells until it manages to break the cells down completely, finally killing them. Radiation accomplishes this, Dr. Tappel suggested, by causing the formation within the cells of so-called free radicals, compounds that careen around the cell, destroying its vital components. The free radicals are formed, Dr. Tappel suggested, when radiation strikes polyunsaturated fats not protected by Vitamin E. An ample supply of vitamin E—enough to maintain adequate levels in the body under any circumstances and certainly an amount sufficient to protect the increased amounts of polyunsaturates we are eating—Tappel said, would protect us against premature free-radical damage. "Continuing research," Tappel suggested, "should more fully explore the possibility that optimization of vitamin E intake may have a deterrent effect on the aging process."

But continuing research has yet to show that vitamin E is the fountain of youth. Certainly, mice fed the substance in abundant quantities have not turned into rodent versions of Methuselah. At a conference on vitamin E, held by the New York Academy of Sciences in 1982, researchers presented evidence that while dietary anti-oxidants can increase the mean and median lifespans of mice, they have not contributed to increasing the animals' maximum lifespans.

Tappel too has hedged his bets. Although in the early 1970s he was enthusiastic about the anti-aging possibilities in vitamin E, by the mid-1970s he was modifying his position somewhat. "Scientists engaged in aging research," Tappel said in the mid-1970s, "have not obtained information to suggest that extra vitamin E might have a positive effect on slowing down aging . . . We cannot be too optimistic that vitamin-E-type anti-oxidants can offer extra protection against any . . . deterioration in the aging process. Apparently, optimum protection is already provided by a nutritious diet, as, for example, by the basic diet fed to control mice [that is, mice not given added amounts of E]."

Researchers like Dr. Tengerdy, Dr. Tappel, and others may, despite setbacks in their attempts to link theory to practice, eventually make important discoveries about vitamin E. But there is no doubt that their research—and research into vitamin E in general— has been drastically affected by those who tout the vitamin as a cure-all, hucksters out to make a quick buck on the vitamin, naïve (or overimaginative, take your choice) doctors who are willing to practice medicine on the basis of what they ardently want to believe is right rather than on the basis of what has been proven to be, beyond a shadow of a doubt, scientifically right.

The vociferous claims made by vitamin E aficionados have, some researchers say, hindered alpha-tocopherol research in two ways. Many researchers who might under different circumstances be avidly pursuing studies of vitamin E are staying away from alpha-tocopherol because they are afraid that any study, no matter how innocently conceived or conservatively and quietly carried out, will immediately land them in bed with the faddists. And rather than take even the slightest chance that they will be tarred by the vitamin enthusiasts' brush, they go on to study something with less potential for controversy. "This group," says one vitamin expert, "has no doubt caused many competent investigators to abjure vitamin E research."

But the wild-eyed faddists cannot be given lone credit for making vitamin E a taboo research area. A fair number of scientists and doctors are so afraid that research into vitamin E's role in any emotionally laden human life process—heart, aging, breathing, reproduction—will just give the lunatic fringe more fuel for its crazy claims that they are quite willing to exert pressure to stop their fellow scientists from venturing into this twilight territory. "When I thought some years ago that vitamin E might be important in slowing down the aging process," Tappel says, "I thought it was important enough to alert our fellow scientists. I sent out about fifty letters, and about half reacted by saying, well, okay. But others approached me and said, 'Boy, that is dangerous ground. You are overextending yourself, you are going to have your financial resources cut off.' They were saying that they would desert us if we persisted. They were putting on pressure."

CHAPTER IV

From Saskatchewan—
An Answer for Schizophrenia

Early in 1952 a seventeen-year-old boy—let's call him Peter—lay dying in the psychiatric ward of Saskatchewan Hospital in Weyburn, a small town tucked away in the southeastern corner of the Canadian province of Saskatchewan. Twenty-three years ago Weyburn had a population of only a few thousand (the vast, sprawling province had less than one million inhabitants). But even in this somewhat rural environment, Peter, who had been diagnosed a schizophrenic, had already received a full range of psychiatric treatments. Electric convulsive therapy—electroshock—had made no inroads against his madness. A series of twenty-four insulin shocks—a treatment, now out of favor, that consists of massive doses of insulin given to produce a temporary coma, which would hopefully interrupt or destroy the aberrant mental processes responsible for bringing on the schizophrenia—had accomplished nothing. In fact, the treatments had left the young man with Bell's palsy, a partial paralysis of the face muscles.

In what were clearly the final stages of his illness, Peter was lashing out viciously at the nurses and attendants trying to look after him, and had to be strapped to his bed. Because he resisted help much of the time, he was wallowing in his own dirt. He had long ago given up food, and only an intravenous solution, dripping slowly through a tube leading to one vein of one arm, hung between him and starvation.

In another part of the psychiatric ward of this prairie hospital a fifty-year-old man was also doing more than his share to keep the already harassed ward staff busy. Daniel (not his real name) had been brought to the hospital shortly after Christmas, 1951. Daniel had always celebrated Christmas with a good drinking bout, and the 1951 season of joy had not been any different. He had celebrated the birth of Jesus Christ with one of his more spectacular sprees; he had drunk for three straight days. In the wake of that nonstop drinking binge, he suddenly found himself sleeping incessantly. When awake, he ate compulsively. He found he had to urinate frequently. He could hardly walk because his legs were so stiff, and when he did walk, he looked like a man teetering along on stilts. Throughout the prolonged hangover in the post-holiday period, he suffered a continually throbbing headache.

His family had already brought him to the hospital once after his Christmas celebration, but he had stayed only a week because he had begun to feel much better. But barely two days after his discharge, he was back at the hospital doors, apparently slipping into insanity. In the hospital, he exposed himself proudly to the nurses and, if they managed to avoid him, he would bare himself to whatever male member of the staff happened to be around. He masturbated publicly. When he tired of both activities, he would find himself an empty chair (or an empty corner of the ward) and would sit there quietly for hours, one finger stuck in a nostril.

As time progressed, Daniel's condition deteriorated. He verbally abused the staff, screaming and shouting at anyone who would cross his path. He paced the halls, up and down, up and down, until he dropped from exhaustion. He took to shedding his clothes, began to have delusions, and soon began to attack physically anyone within easy reach.

Having tried everything else, convinced that both Peter and Daniel were on the road to complete self-destruction, Dr. Abram Hoffer, at the time director of psychiatric research in Saskatchewan's Department of Public Health, and Humphrey Osmond, clinical director of the Saskatchewan Hospital, decided that this was the right opportunity to test their theory that nicotinic acid in massive doses might be useful in combating mental illness, particularly schizophrenia. Peter was the first to be given the vitamin in huge quantities. "He was given a combination of 10 Gm of nicotinic acid and 5 Gm of ascorbic acid daily in two divided dosages,'' the two Canadian researchers reported in 1957 in the *Journal of Clinical and Experimental Psychopathology.* "The first day these were given in a solution by tube. The second day the patient was able to bring the glass to his lips and drink the medication. At the end of thirty days, this man was completely well.''

Daniel, Hoffer and Osmond reported, responded just as well when they treated him with nicotinic acid. "He was given 3 Gm of nicotinamide [an alternative form of nicotinic acid] per day,'' they wrote. "Two days later, the patient was greatly improved and was able to participate in a rational conversation. The following day, the patient was relatively well. Treatment was continued for one month, and the patient was discharged one month after that.''

Schizophrenia is one of the major psychiatric problems challenging medicine today. It is a distressing disease because its victims are by and large young people, men and women in their late teens, twenties, and early thirties. It is a devastating disease. A few patients—no more than 30 percent—recover from their first bout with schizophrenia and stay well for the rest of their lives. But the other 70 percent suffer through recurring bouts of schizophrenia. They spend the rest of their lives checking in and out of hospital mental wards, lying around at home under heavy sedation, waiting and hoping for a remission that will give them an opportunity to lead normal lives at least part of the time. A host of treatments—insulin shock therapy, electroshock therapy, camphor in oil injections to produce convulsions, psychotherapy, behavior-modification therapy in which rewards and punishments are used systematically to try to change the schizophrenic's behavior patterns—have accomplished little or nothing either in diminishing the incidence of schizophrenia or in lessening its iron grip on 70 percent of its victims.

In Canada about one half of all the beds in mental hospitals in the psychiatric wards of general hospitals are occupied by people in the throes of schizophrenia. In the United States nearly two million persons suffer from the disease. In 1969 almost 70 percent of all the people admitted to state and county mental hospitals in the United States were schizophrenics who had received care in these institutions before. One fifth of those who are hospitalized with schizophrenia spend years, not months, in bolted and locked wards.

Little progress has been made against the disease because since the day schizophrenia was identified and baptized in 1899 it has been, in the words of Dr. J. D. Griffin, general director of the Canadian Mental Health Association, "a psychiatric enigma and a virtually unresolved problem for modern medicine." Some of the enigma is rooted in the fact that the disease is extremely difficult to diagnose. Much of the mystery remains simply because researchers cannot find or agree on the cause or causes of schizophrenia.

Although the word *schizophrenia* is freely tossed about by professional and layman alike, psychiatrists often disagree on diagnoses of schizophrenia and have a difficult time deciding which patient is schizophrenic and which is not. The disease, many psychiatrists say, is a complex one, a tricky slippery illness on which to pin a hard-and-fast diagnostic label. Even batteries of assorted tests, careful observations by psychiatrists, psychologists, and trained nurses, all compiled and collated, do not make it easy to arrive at a certain diagnosis. Psychiatrists often find that they have to change their diagnosis of a particular patient after they have stamped SCHIZOPHRENIA across his chart. One researcher, looking into diagnosis problems, found that only 37 percent of the patients who had been diagnosed as schizophrenic at their first hospitalization retained that label by the time they had been institutionalized a fourth time. Another psychiatric researcher found that even the nationality and locality of the psychiatrist will influence the label that a psychiatrist will pin on a mentally ill person. The researcher showed video tapes of interviews with emotionally disturbed persons to psychiatrists in London and New York, and on the West Coast. At various times during the interview, patients showed an inability to organize their thoughts. They showed tremendous swings in mood. The New York psychiatrists, weighing heavily the ability to organize thinking, said the patients were schizophrenic because they were unable to give clear direction to their thoughts. The London psychiatrists, more impressed by the ups and downs in the patients' moods, said that they were manic-depressive. When the West Coast psychiatrists saw the same tapes, their diagnoses agreed with those of their colleagues in London, not with those of their colleagues in New York.

In much the same way, schizophrenia taunts doctors because

scientists have yet to come up with a satisfactory explanation for the origins of the disease.

Some researchers argue that schizophrenia is a hereditary disease, passed on from generation to generation through the transmission of faulty genetic material. That schizophrenia often appears in subsequent generations of the same family, some genetically oriented psychiatrists argue, bears out the hereditary explanation for the appearance of schizophrenia. Those who subscribe to this school of thought also point out that studies conducted with twins yield strong evidence to back up a theory for schizophrenia based on genetics. When identical twins—twins that carry identical genetic material because they develop from the same egg, fertilized by the same sperm—are studied, these geneticists say, if one twin develops schizophrenia, the chances are good, as high as 75 percent, that the other one will develop the disease as well. On the other hand, it is pointed out, when fraternal twins—twins that carry dissimilar genetic material because they are born from two different eggs, fertilized by two different sperm—are studied statistically, it appears that the chances that both will develop schizophrenia are as low as one in fifteen.

There are other schizophrenia experts who argue that the genetic theory is nonsense, that it is the child's environment that determines whether or not he will develop the disease. If a child develops schizophrenia in a household in which one parent or both parents are schizophrenic, it is because the child has "learned" the disease. Constantly exposed to an ambient schizophrenia, the child in time is beaten down by the disease as well.

Still another group of theoreticians offers another hypothesis. Neither genetics nor environment alone set off schizophrenic symptoms, this viewpoint holds, but, rather, the disease is a result of interaction between genes and environment. The individual who turns schizophrenic does not carry within him one gene (or set of genes) that suddenly brings on mental illness. Instead, that person probably carries a genetic heritage for schizophrenia that lies dormant until something comes along to rouse the genetic predisposition into action.

To take an example from another branch of medicine: a person may be born with a genetic deficiency that does not allow the metabolic processes in the body to break down ingested fats properly.

That is, there might be something wrong with the genes that control the production of those enzymes that play an important role in breaking down, converting, and utilizing some fats (usually so-called saturated fats) present in food. Instead of being used to advantage in the body, instead of being shunted, in greatly simplified form into systems that would excrete them from the body, the fats are allowed to linger in the body, to accumulate in the walls of key arteries until they plug the vessels and set off a heart attack or a stroke. In some similar fashion (although the exact processes are not understood), some researchers believe, the environment and the genes conspire to bring on attacks of schizophrenia in some people. Studies that show that children of schizophrenic parents are less likely—though not completely unlikely—to develop schizophrenia if they are raised in an adoptive home where the adults are mentally stable are often cited as support for this point of view.

Finally, just as many researchers scorn the theories that heredity or environmental stresses (or both) can cause schizophrenia. They argue instead that aberrant biochemical processes in the body are responsible for the disease, although they cannot satisfactorily or completely explain what those processes might be, how they do their debilitating work, or where in the brain they do it. Some researchers have found that blood samples taken from psychotics have an abnormally high amount of an enzyme produced by muscle tissue, an enzyme called creatine phosphokinase. Other researchers have found a mysterious link between histamines—the same compounds that dilate blood vessels, reduce blood pressure, and stimulate gastric secretions—and mental illnesses like schizophrenia. Some of the studies have demonstrated that people whose mental troubles include paranoia and hallucinations have low levels of histamine in their blood, while those who have serious depressions have high histamine levels. No one has yet to offer any widely accepted theory explaining the meaning of these findings.

In an effort to bring some unity to the schizophrenia research community, some suggest a kind of a compromise. It is altogether possible, these consensus theoreticians say, that schizophrenia is not really a single disease, that, rather, it is a symptom of many different diseases and bodily malfunctions. A cough, for example, may signal a simple chest cold, pneumonia, tuberculosis, emphysema, cancer, or asthma, to name a few respiratory diseases. The cough, however, always sounds more or less the same. In much the same way, some researchers say, any given schizophrenic episode might have any one of a number of roots and could be the manifestation of any one of a number of processes. Thus, some researchers suggest, it might be worthwhile to try to sort out the different causes of schizophrenia and to concentrate on finding different cures for each one. These attempts at compromise, however, don't go very far. "On one end of this campus there are the psychiatrists who claim that schizophrenia is strictly a psychogenic condition due to an abnormal mother-child relationship," Dr. Bernard Kaufman sums up. "On the other end of the campus there are biochemists who claim that schizophrenia is a biochemical deficiency in the brain, that there are vital compounds missing. You bring these two groups together in one room and all hell breaks loose."

Just about the only ones who feel that there is nothing to argue about in discussing schizophrenia are vitamin enthusiasts. They believe that schizophrenia is indeed a disease with biochemical roots, but that the vitamin nicotinic acid (or niacin, the name preferred by those who don't like the unfortunate implication that the vitamin is exclusively involved with tobacco, the plant in which it was first isolated) applied in massive doses will help the patient live a substantially normal life.

Much of the enthusiasm for nicotinic acid's alleged effectiveness against schizophrenia is rooted in the experiences early vitamin and nutrition researchers had in using the vitamin to eradicate pellagra around the turn of the century. Pellagra is characterized in scientific shorthand by the four D's—diarrhea, dermatitis, dementia, death. The pellagrin (as pellagra sufferers are called) has skin that looks sunburned. The disease is also distinguished by skin inflammations that turn to blisters. Often the blisters become infected. In pellagra the lining of the mouth becomes sore, red, and highly sensitive to hot or spicy foods. The tongue swells and reddens and sometimes becomes ulcerated. The patient has periods of constipation that alternate with diarrhea. As the disease progresses, the sufferer becomes apprehensive, irritable, forgetful, and paranoid. In time a full-blown psychosis sets in. And ultimately, if the disease is left untreated, the patient dies.

In the first two decades of the century, mental hospitals in the southern United States were filled with patients in advanced stages of pellagra. (The disease, nutritionists now know, establishes a vicious circle. The pellagrin develops psychotic tendencies because of the disease. Then, because he is psychotic and has strange fantasies and fears about the food he is given, he refuses to eat or develops bizarre food consumption patterns. They in turn aggravate or perpetuate the pellagra.) In fact, in the first two decades of this century, there were between 100,000 and 200,000 cases of pellagra reported in the United States, mostly in the South, where its victims had been living on maize meal, molasses, and meat, usually salt pork. In South Carolina, Mississippi, and Alabama, pellagra was among the five leading causes of death.

Because the disease was so prevalent among blacks and poor whites, established opinion at the turn of the century had it that pellagra was due to bad hygiene. A few nutrition experts, including notably Dr. Joseph Goldberger of the U.S. Public Health Service, thought not. The disease, Goldberger felt, was probably due to some nutritional deficiency. To prove his point, Goldberger obtained permission to carry out an experiment in two southern orphanages and a lunatic asylum where there had been extensive outbreaks of pellagra. Goldberger changed the diets on which the experimental subjects had been living, giving them greater variety of meat, vegetables, and fruits, as well as eggs. No one who at the beginning of the experiment did not have pellagra developed the disease. Two hundred subjects who did have pellagra when the experiment began recovered on the improved diet.

To find further proof that the disease was rooted in poor nutrition, Goldberger placed eleven convicts (who were promised pardons in exchange for their cooperation in the experiment) on diets similar to those eaten by poor people in Mississippi, where the disease was endemic. Of the eleven convicts who participated in the experiment, five developed pellagra. Despite the proof Goldberger was amassing, many nutritionists and public-health experts of the day still insisted that the disease was caused by some sort of an infective process that was caused by dirty living habits. To still the opposition finally, Goldberger undertook the ultimate experiment: he and fifteen researchers who had been working with him tried to give themselves pellagra by infecting themselves with a mixture that was composed of blood, nasal secretions, feces, and urine taken from sufferers of pellagra. None of the researchers developed the disease.

It took almost another two decades to isolate the factor—a new vitamin that was called nicotinic acid—in Goldberger's improved diet that was eradicating pellagra. But almost as soon as the final results of Goldberger's experiments were in, diets in asylums around the South were improved. One result was that thousands of inmates who had shown severe emotional disturbances suddenly recovered their senses enough to be released.

The fact that pellagra was accompanied by mental aberrations resembling those of schizophrenia—changes in personality, delusions, visions, changes in taste and smell, hallucinations—and that the pellagra-related personality changes could be eradicated by simply giving the pellagrin a small daily amount of nicotinic acid impressed some latter-day psychiatrists who were working with schizophrenics. Among those who were to be most impressed with the potential usefulness of nicotinic acid in the treatment of mental illness was Dr. Hoffer.

Hoffer's quest for biochemical roots and biochemical solutions for schizophrenia actually began in the early 1950s—before Peter and Daniel were admitted to the psychiatric ward of Saskatchewan Hospital. Hoffer and Osmond had begun their search because they had noted that mescaline, when given experimentally to research subjects or when taken by drug addicts in search of a high, often brought about the same behavior patterns and the same symptoms observed in schizophrenia. Hoffer and Osmond were also intrigued by the fact that mescaline and adrenaline are close chemical cousins. Adrenaline occurs naturally in the body. It is a hormone that is secreted judiciously by the adrenal glands to regulate a wide assortment of functions, including the body's responses to various stresses. In time of danger, adrenaline pours into the bloodstream causing the heart to pump faster and move blood, with its essential load of oxygen and nutrients, around the body faster to stoke the muscles with energy needed to meet danger. But adrenaline, in and of itself, does not produce hallucinations or other psychological disturbances. And mescaline, Hoffer and Osmond knew, while it does produce psychological changes, does not occur naturally in the body. Could it be, Hoffer and Osmond asked themselves, that some other substance lying on the chemical continuum with adrenaline and mescaline, a substance somehow related to them both, could be produced in the body? Could the body perhaps be using some of the component parts of adrenaline and be turning them into a mescalinelike substance? Could this aberrant by-product be causing the schizophrenia?

In discussing their ideas with colleagues in Saskatchewan, Dr, Hoffer and Osmond found encouragement to pursue their theory. They learned that during the Second World War, anesthetists, who use adrenaline during the anesthesia procedure, were often hampered by supply shortages and had to use supplies of adrenaline that had been stored on hospital shelves too long. Patients who were given this old adrenaline, one anesthetist told Hoffer and Osmond, often displayed bizarre psychological problems. Chemists, they also learned, had determined that the adrenaline, left too long on the shelf, had deteriorated and had turned into another chemical called adrenochrome. Others told Hoffer and Osmond that some patients given adrenaline shots to control asthma attacks or allergy attacks also sometimes suffered transient episodes of emotional instability.

Pursuing these various hints, Hoffer and Osmond (and a third researcher named John Smythies) established that adrenochrome, like adrenaline, shared many chemical characteristics with hallucinogens like mescaline. And, although they had no proof that adrenochrome could be manufactured by the body (and there is still no proof of that), the Canadian researchers came to be convinced that a bodily form of shelf adrenochrome was in fact responsible for schizophrenia. To prove to themselves that the substance could be responsible for the disease, Dr. Hoffer and Osmond—as well as their wives and one other volunteer—took doses of the chemical and observed each other's (and their own) reactions to it. "My experiences in the laboratory were on the whole pleasant but when I left I found the corridors outside sinister and unfriendly," Osmond wrote later in recording his "trips" on adrenochrome. ". . . I began to wonder whether I was a person any more and to think that I might be a plant or stone. As my feeling for these inanimate objects increased, my feeling for and my interest in humans diminished. I felt indifferent towards humans and had to curb myself from making unpleasant personal remarks about them."

Although there was no proof for the presence of adrenochrome in the human body, the Canadians thought they could fashion a good theoretical framework to explain its role in schizophrenia. In every human being, they reasoned, adrenaline and its precursors (substances used by the body to manufacture the adrenaline itself) are constantly being changed into different compounds. When the process works as it should, the reshuffling of the chemicals, the theory went, proceeds along orderly fashion with all of the usual products and by-products going off to do their specific jobs in various parts of the body. But in someone with schizophrenia, Hoffer and Osmond proposed, the process has somehow gone wrong. Chemicals that should not be added or should not be part of the adrenaline process find themselves attached to adrenaline by-products. The interference of the wrong chemical, they concluded, made for the appearance of a hallucinogenic compound, namely, adrenochrome.

The key question, of course, was how they could abort the aberrant process, how to stop these "wrong" chemicals from subverting adrenaline and bringing on the apprearance of the theoretical adrenochrome. It occurred to Hoffer and Osmond that perhaps some other substance could be used to interfere with the schizophrenia-inducing process, some substance that would in the body attract and neutralize the chemicals that were helping in the manufacture of adrenochrome. Because they were familiar with the chemical composition of nicotinic acid, Hoffer, Osmond, and Smythies reasoned that, in massive doses, the vitamin could compete for, attract, and get out of the way the chemicals responsible for the formation of adrenochrome. On the whole the reasoning was somewhat inaccurate: neither the Hoffer team, nor any other research team, had actually isolated adrenochrome in the human body.

In time, Hoffer's view of the chemical processes involved in the disease changed. By the 1960s he was still arguing that there was some malfunction in the transformation of chemicals that controlled psychological balance within the brain. But now he switched his focus of attention away from aberrations in adrenaline production to aberrations in the supply of vitamin-related substances. In 1966 Hoffer and Osmond suggested that a compound called nicotinamide adenine dinucleotide (NAD, for short) was essential to the proper functioning of the brain. Since NAD is a nicotinic-acid derivative, they said, all of us need a good supply of the vitamin to maintain proper brain function. Without nicotinic acid, without NAD, we would turn schizophrenic, no less psychotic then the hapless inmates of southern insane asylums at the beginning of the 1900s. But in some other people, Hoffer and Osmond suggested, a normal supply of nicotinic acid is not enough to ward off schizophrenia. In these certain people, a metabolic error, perhaps of genetic origin, blocks the delivery of proper amounts of NAD to the brain. In these people only massive amounts of nicotinic acid, enough to overpower whatever it is that stood in the way of proper NAD delivery to the brain, could abort schizophrenic episodes.

Hoffer and Osmond began presenting evidence in support of their theories that nicotinic acid is effective against schizophrenia in the mid-1950s with a report in the 1957 April–June issue of the *Journal of Clinical and Experimental Psychopathology*. After Peter and Daniel had responded in encouraging fashion to massive doses of nicotinic acid, Dr. Hoffer's research team reported, thirty patients were chosen to participate in further studies of nicotinic acid. Nine patients were given a placebo, an inactive preparation that has no pharmacological effect but leads the patient to believe that he is getting a ''new'' medicine; ten patients were given nicotinic acid; eleven were given nicotinamide. Some patients in each group were also given electric convulsive therapy. The study lasted six weeks: one week at the beginning to evaluate the mental state of the patients, four weeks of treatment, one week to assess the results of the treatment. When the results of the study had been compiled, Dr. Hoffer and Osmond reported, it was obvious that the vitamin had had a significant impact. ''The patients receiving the placebo had remained well one-third of the time,'' the Canadians reported, ''whereas the other two groups of patients remained well two-thirds of the time.''

For the next several years, Dr. Hoffer and his associates continued their work with nicotinic acid, treating selected groups of patients with massive doses of the vitamin, and comparing the course of their disease with the course of schizophrenia in patients who were being treated with more conventional methods. Thus, in a 1964 article, after analyzing the fate of various schizophrenia patients over a ten-year span, Dr. Hoffer reported that ''when newly-admitted schizophrenics are given nicotinic acid treatment of the kind we have used, far more of them remain well than with other treatments presently in use.''

Typical of the patients who had benefited from nicotinic acid therapy, Hoffer and Osmond reported in their 1964 article, was a man—they called him P.F. to protect his identity—who was brought to the hospital because his father was worried about his strange behavior. Mr. P.F. had become convinced that people in his community were constantly picking on him (he had even filed a complaint against his neighbors with the local police). He harbored suspicions suddenly that his wife had been unfaithful to him and that his children had been fathered by other men.

Mr. P.F.'s greatest problem was that he had, just before his hospitalization, become increasingly obsessed with his World War II experiences. He convinced himself that he was responsible for the failure of the Allied expedition against the German troops sur-rounding the French port of Dieppe. P.F. told his psychiatrists that during the war he and three friends who were on patrol had wandered too close to German lines. The Germans had spotted the group and had begun firing. P.F. and his friends split up, he and one buddy running to the right, the other two running to the left. He and his companion, who was shot in the leg, escaped. But the other two soldiers were killed. Later in the war P.F. was badly wounded by shrapnel in Holland and was given an honorable discharge. He returned to Canada, married, and settled down to a life of farming.

Mr. P.F. was convinced that the ill-fated patrol in which he had participated had alerted the German command to Allied plans. Later, he became convinced that his two friends had not really been killed in the confrontation with the Germans and that the whole scene had been staged to test him in some way. P.F. found an official history of his regiment and read through it. In it he found the two men listed as dead. That, however, did not satisfy him—and he came to the conclusion that this particular section in the regimental history had been rewritten to further the conspiracy against him.

After three weeks on nicotinic acid, Hoffer and Osmond wrote, P.F. improved, his delusions faded, and he was released. A year later he was still well. ''His wife was severely ill in hospital, but he had handled the very difficult stressful situation well,'' Hoffer and

Osmond said. "All his delusions were gone. . . . He was operating his farm efficiently, led an active social life, and got on well with his neighbors."

All in all, Hoffer and Osmond wrote in 1964, the patients who had received nicotinic acid as far back as 1952 had fared far better in the decade lapsing 1952 and 1962 than patients who had not received the vitamin but who had been treated with conventional psychiatric methods. That the patients who had received nicotinic acid had apparently done well was especially gratifying, Hoffer and Osmond said, because the patients who had received the vitamin regimen had been those who had been at the bottom of the psychiatric barrel. Other psychiatrists associated with the hospital where Hoffer and Osmond conducted their work had agreed to let only their worst patients, the ones who had shown no response whatsoever to other treatment modalities, enter the experiments with nicotinic acid. "We hoped at first to get every patient from the ward who was diagnosed schizophrenic," Hoffer and Osmond said, "but this more satisfactory design was not possible because the psychiatric staff who were neither engaged in research or [sic] well disposed towards it, did not want their best patients included in it." [1]

The patients on nicotinic acid, Hoffer and Osmond reported, fared significantly better than a comparison group of patients who did not receive the vitamin. "Twelve out of sixteen or 75 per cent of the nicotinic acid group did not require readmissions [to a mental hospital] for ten years, i.e., there has been a 75 percent cure rate," Hoffer and Osmond reported. In contrast they said, they could report that only ten of twenty-seven—or a comparatively low 36 percent—of the comparison group were still well after ten years.

As part of their study, Hoffer and Osmond calculated how much time nicotinic acid patients had spent in hospitals over the previous ten years. Hoffer and Osmond found that 76 patients who

---

[1] This proud assertion is particularly significant. When later experiments by other researchers failed to duplicate the claims made by many orthomolecular psychiatrists, the orthomolecularists argued that the regimen had not worked in the hands of skeptics because the skeptics had chosen schizophrenics whose illness was too far advanced or had treated very seriously ill schizophrenics with an inadequate megavitamin therapy. Early in his claims, however, Dr. Hoffer maintained that even the sickest patients responded to his treatment. Moreover, his early prescriptions for schizophrenia were relatively modest in their use of nicotinic acid and/or ancillary vitamins and other psychiatric procedures.

had been diagnosed as schizophrenic and who had received nicotinic acid had spent a collective 2,453 days in the hospital over the seven-year period—an average of about 5 days per patient per year. On the other hand, Hoffer and Osmond said, 226 patients who were diagnosed as schizophrenic and were treated only with standard tranquilizers, ECT, and psychotherapy required 25,341 days of hospitalization, or about 16 days per patient per year.

According to the Canadians, the nicotinic acid also succeeded in cutting down suicides. Five out of 348 patients who did not get nicotinic acid, Hoffer and Osmond said, killed themselves—a rate of 1.47 per 100 patients over the seven-year period they had studied. None of the patients who had received massive doses of nicotinic acid had killed themselves in the same seven-year period. "One could conclude that not giving schizophrenic patients nicotinic acid as part of an overall treatment program as we have described it, exposes every 100,000 patients to a risk that 220 will commit suicide," Hoffer and Osmond wrote.

"There can be no reason why massive nicotinic acid should not alter the outcome in schizophrenia," Hoffer and Osmond concluded. "Apart from deep prejudice or sheer inertia, it is worth trying because it meets one of the major requirements of any treatment, that of 'doing no harm.' Two-thirds of those who develop schizophrenia are more or less crippled by it and return to hospital for periods ranging from a few weeks to several years. . . . We think that these young people, who are doomed to be in and out of mental hospitals for most of their lives, have a right to be given nicotinic acid even if medical men are sceptical."

The aged, suffering the psychoses of old age, could also be helped by the vitamin, Hoffer said. "I have seen patients around age 70, take nicotinic acid regularly for ten years and during this period there has been no senile deterioration," Dr. Hoffer wrote in *Diseases of the Nervous System* in June, 1965. "These patients are alert, clear minded and active as if there has been no further mental aging. Several had shown clear senile changes when the vitamin was started ten years ago. These symptoms were reversed within a few days after the nicotinic acid was started."

Even a seventy-three-year-old man struggling against terminal cancer and struck by what he diagnosed as schizophrenia, Hoffer wrote in that 1965 article, had been helped by massive doses of nicotinic acid. He had entered University Hospital in Saskatoon because he had been deteriorating physically. Doctors discovered lung cancer. Shortly after the diagnosis, the man grew depressed, irrational, and confused. His doctors first thought that his depression was a natural reaction to the illness. But as changes in his personality became more radical, they came to think that the malignancy had spread to the brain. He was transferred to the psychiatric ward, where he began suffering hallucinations.

Dr. Hoffer discovered that the man's urine samples contained a compound—Dr. Hoffer calls it the mauve factor—which he believes is produced in the bodies of schizophrenics and which can be taken as a sure sign that the mental aberrations exhibited by a patient are indeed schizophrenia. Convinced that the man's mental problems were of a schizophrenic, not cancerous, nature, Dr. Hoffer gave him three grams of nicotinic acid and three grams of ascorbic acid a day. "The patient . . . was discharged clinically nearly normal in four days," Dr. Hoffer reported. "Six months after discharge he has remained mentally normal, and, according to one informant, a physician and close friend of his, he is better than he has been in several years. He continues to take both medicines regularly. After fifteen months, he is still normal."

To Dr. Hoffer's astonishment—and disappointment—his flood of reports and articles out of Saskatoon had little impact on the psychiatric world. There were no cheers of approval. There weren't (at first) even many jeers of disapproval. The major tranquilizers—tranquilizers we know today as Thorazine, Stelazine, Valium—had only recently been introduced to the psychiatric community with a good deal of fanfare. And, while these new drugs were not curing schizophrenia, they were proving to be effective in controlling some of the symptoms of the disease sufficiently to allow many schizophrenics to leave mental hospitals and to live at home. Almost no one in the medical community was inclined to listen to claims that mere vitamins could be equally—if not more—effective against this devastating disease.

If the news out of Canada did not bring the medical and scientific communities to their feet cheering, it did impress a vast number of lay people and an adventurous psychiatrist here and there who had read the Hoffer reports in the various journals.

Alcoholics were among those who were the first to turn to massive doses of nicotinic acid for help. Many alcoholics are schizophrenics (and vice versa), and the reports of the vitamin's alleged effectiveness against the mental illness drew their attention. Moreover, alcoholics (even those who are not schizophrenic) often suffer severe depressions, especially when they abstain from drink, and many former drinkers began to look to the vitamin to help them withstand the shock of the psychological potholes along the road to permanent sobriety. In fact, alcoholics have been among the most fervent of proselytizers for nicotinic acid. When one Texas alcoholic found that the vitamin seemed to help him with his problems, he prepared one thousand letters describing the virtues of nicotinic acid and mailed them out to many psychiatrists and alcoholics in his town. "About eighteen months ago I spoke to an AA friend in New York who endured years of acute depression," another reformed alcoholic said recently. "[Nicotinic acid] completely relieved his condition. He began to recommend the vitamin in semiorganized fashion by actively seeking out fellow AA sufferers. They in turn described the benefits they received to still others. In consequence, my friend now estimates that some four hundred people in his vicinity are using [nicotinic acid]."

The ardor with which the word about nicotinic acid was spread by nonprofessionals was soon evident to anyone charting vitamin sales in pharmaceutical houses. In the first half of 1966, for example, one wholesaler on the East Coast received only 31 orders for bottles containing 500-milligram nicotinic acid pills, and of these orders, only three were from doctors. By the time 1966 had ended, this wholesaler had received 652 orders for nicotinic acid pills—and 25 percent of the orders came from physicians, presumably the very few doctors who had been convinced of the vitamin's effectiveness.

Among those physicians impressed by what alcoholics and former alcoholics had to say was Dr. David Hawkins, director of the North Nassau Mental Health Center in Manhasset, New York.

When the center first opened its doors in 1956, it treated patients with conventional methods of the day and continued doing so until 1965, when a member of Alcoholics Anonymous who had links to the center suggested that Dr. Hawkins try this new application for nicotinic acid on a group of twenty-four schizophrenics who had formed a Schizophrenics Anonymous group at Fordham University.

Impressed by the preliminary results, Hawkins began to use the vitamin more and more. In the 1960s Dr. Hawkins conducted a study with 160 patients—94 women and 66 men—who had been diagnosed as schizophrenic and who had been under treatment at the Brunswick Hospital in Amityville, Long Island. During their stay in the hospital, all the patients received regular daily doses of a tranquilizer, 50 milligrams of vitamin B_6 (pyridoxine), 4 grams of ascorbic acid, and 4 to 10 grams of nicotinic acid or nicotinamide. Upon discharge, Hawkins said, 85 of the patients were taken off the vitamin regimen. The rest were divided into groups that received the megavitamins for three months, six months, and one year after they left the hospital. During the year following discharge, Dr. Hawkins reported in the journal *Psychosomatics,* 30 patients—35 percent of the total—who did not receive megavitamins were rehospitalized. Only 25 percent of the patients who took vitamins for three to ten months had to be rehospitalized within one year. Of the 57 patients who were faithful to their vitamins for one year or more, only 9—16 percent—were rehospitalized. "This study," Dr. Hawkins summarized, "establishes a definite correlation between the continuation of megavitamin therapy and a 50 percent lower readmission rate than patients in the control group."

Dr. Hawkins became a firm believer in megavitamin treatment. With Dr. Pauling, he co-edited a 700-page book on the subject of vitamin treatment of mental disease, *Orthomolecular Psychiatry: Treatment of Schizophrenia.* The interview I conduct with him takes place in his warmly decorated office, subtly lit, graced with a stained glass window. It is obvious as we chat that he is a busy man. Patients come to him for as far away as Alaska, New Caledonia, Venezuela. He supervises the center's links to a hospital, a halfway house for patients released from the hospital, a Schizophrenics Anonymous group, and a family service center.

Dr. Hawkins, a small man, nattily dressed, talks almost detachedly about his vitamin experiences. They are, after all, routine medication now, beyond discussion or debate, as far as he is concerned. "What we had heard about megavitamins seemed preposterous and outrageous,'' he says quietly. ''But we tried them and the results astounded us.''

It is a cold late-November day, and a steady drizzle hits the sides of the colonial-style building where the center is housed. The window in the small office is open, but somehow the cold doesn't seem to penetrate. Dr. Hawkins, pondering the many patients who have come to him, leans back in his chair, tilting it on its hind legs, pressing his fingertips against the edge of his desk for balance.

''Schizophrenia,'' he says, keeping his voice down as if not to disturb what ghosts those patients who have come through here might have left behind, ''is a formidable disease. When you deal with it, you are dealing with an illness that destroys a life. You hate to withhold anything that might have a margin of help in it.

''I just had a patient here who had been sick for four years. Three of those years she had spent in a psychoanalytic-type therapy. And, after this treatment by well-known names in the field at a cost of a quarter of a million dollars, she came here mute, catatonic. She had lost one fourth of her weight and was slowly dying of starvation. She wouldn't take food or medication. She would just stand in the middle of the room and not move. Now, exactly two weeks after treatment was begun, here she is walking around normally, talking, taking her medication. We'll discharge her within eight weeks.''

By 1968 a few psychiatrists here and there had been converted to the nicotinic acid cause. Hundreds of laymen, seeking help for mental problems and dissatisfied with the treatments they had been given by members of the more conventional psychiatric establishment, were seeking out those practitioners who believed in nicotinic acid and megavitamin therapy. But all in all, the nicotinic acid movement seemed doomed to crawl along in relative obscurity. But in 1968 the spotlight suddenly swerved, engulfing the megavitamin field in a radiant light, and the source for that light was none other than Linus Pauling, the eminent researcher who towered above American science.

Pauling's entrance into the megavitamin field was a matter of no small importance. He had long ago established himself as one of the world's foremost scientists, the dean of chemistry whose insights into the workings of chemical compounds and whose understanding of chemical principles had been brilliant trailblazers. Like many other people who feel they have gone as far as they can in one field and who seek out other horizons to conquer, Pauling had, late in his career, left chemistry behind to concentrate on the study of human molecular biology. Characteristically, his contributions to this field of endeavor were as brilliant as those he had made in chemistry.

Pauling's efforts to understand biological functions at the molecular level encouraged him to formulate a new theory: disturbances in the molecular environment of the brain—disturbances brought on by a change in the food supply available to man or by a genetic inability to use a particular nutrient efficiently even if it was available—was responsible for a good many of the mental illnesses of man. Brain and nerve tissues are so sensitive to changes in their molecular environment, he argued, that psychological problems could arise long before there were physiological disturbances apparent elsewhere in the body as a result of molecular problems. In fact, Pauling went on, disturbances in the molecular environment in the body might be limited to just one organ, perhaps just the brain. "There is the possibility," Professor Pauling proposed, "that some human beings have a sort of cerebral scurvy, without any of the other manifestations, or a sort of cerebral pellagra, or cerebral pernicious anemia." The judicious application of massive doses of vitamins, Pauling suggested, could be instrumental in reestablishing a correct molecular environment for the brain, and thus could be instrumental in alleviating mental suffering. "The reported success in treating schizophrenia and other mental illnesses by the use of massive doses of some of these vitamins," he wrote in *Science,* "may be the result of successful treatment of a localized cerebral deficiency disease involving the vital substances. . . ."

Pauling's beliefs were all theory. He had no proof that disturbances in the molecular environment of the brain did cause emotional upheavals. He had no proof that the disturbances in the molecular environment even existed. He had only bits and pieces of information to sustain his theoretical musings. And, while it is one thing to bandy about a theory over a cup of coffee in the lounge of the chemistry department, it is quite another to urge that medicine be practiced on the basis of a theory yet to gain proper confirmation.

Pauling's friends and admirers were aghast—and rightly so— that this great man would urge the practice of theoretical medicine with massive doses of substances whose workings—positive or negative—in the human body had never been properly outlined. Nevertheless, by 1971 Pauling had become even more convinced that massive doses of vitamins could be useful in changing the molecular environment of the brain and in curing schizophrenia. "It is the duty of every psychiatrist to add megavitamin therapy to his armamentarium and to make use of these vitamins," Pauling told a meeting of the American Schizophrenia Association in 1971. "To try them out in proper amounts, not just doubling the recommended daily allowance, but in the proper amounts as discussed by Dr. Hoffer and others. . . ."

In embracing the megavitamin approach to schizophrenia, Dr. Pauling did more than just give the movement some scientific responsibility. He even suggested a name: orthomolecular psychiatry, the branch of medicine concerned with achieving an optimum molecular balance in the brain. The title was immediately adopted by psychiatrists who practice megavitamin therapy. In short order, a Society for Orthomolecular Psychiatry was formed, a journal was started to give those practicing in the field a medium of communication, and symposia were organized to bring advocates of the orthomolecular approach together in orderly fashion to discuss and exchange ideas.

In this heady new atmosphere, psychiatrists who had been adding their own innovations to the megavitamin approach now found wider audiences (wider than those they could find in those days when exchange of ideas came largely through phone calls, letters, or chance meetings). In the early years Dr. Hoffer had talked almost exclusively about nicotinic acid. Sometimes he mentioned ascorbic acid, but only in passing. But because depression is often a factor in scurvy, because there were reports that schizophrenics seemed to use up ascorbic acid faster than normal people, and because ascorbic acid was thought to be an important part of the process involved in proper utilization of nicotinic acid, vitamin C was often included in the nicotinic acid regimen for schizophrenics. For similar reasons, others suggested that other vitamins, including E, riboflavin, pyridoxine, and calcium pantothenate, also be included in the megavitamin therapy.

At the same time, many orthomolecular psychiatrists spread the word that in their experience hypoglycemia—low blood sugar—plays a significant role in schizophrenia. Hypoglycemia, with its attendant fatigue, weakness, headaches, irregular heartbeats, dizziness, trembling, cold sweats, excessive hunger bouts, and depressions, could be a significant affliction for anyone unlucky enough to develop it. But, said those who had treated hypoglycemia, when the disease occurs in schizophrenics, the results could be devastating. In fact, they added, hypoglycemia can be detected in up to 70 percent of all schizophrenics, is responsible for attenuating existing schizophrenic symptoms, and is often behind the suicidal urges that kill many of these mentally disturbed men and women. Schizophrenics who were receiving massive doses of vitamins, it was suggested, should also be placed on a hypoglycemic diet, a diet that leads to a proper balance of sugar in the blood, a diet that excludes white-flour products, starches, and sugars, that includes foods high in protein and low in saturated fats, and that makes ample use of fruits and vegetables.

With Pauling's theoretical battle cry to lead the way, and the many new weapons in its armamentarium, the movement was on its way.

CHAPTER V

The Greening of Nicotinic Acid

The galvanization of isolated psychiatrists who had been alone in their faith in nicotinic acid and other vitamins into a well-organized movement gave orthomolecular psychiatry a base (of sorts) within the medical world. Much of that world was still skeptical, if not plainly and increasingly hostile, to the vitamin therapies for mental illness. But the fervor that accompanied the emergence of orthomolecular psychiatry as a well-defined specialty in the wake of Pauling's entrance into the field made for an atmosphere in which more and more doctors who had become dissatisfied with more mundane forms of therapy could switch allegiances and take up the banner of megavitamin therapy without worrying that they had left the fold of respectable medicine.

Dr. William Weathers, head of the San Bernardino County General Hospital Mental Health Unit, in California, began a pilot program to test megavitamin therapy in 1971. But as word of the program spread, the Mental Health Unit began to treat schizophrenics who came seeking megavitamin therapy, but with none of the restraints that might have marked an experimental pilot program.

I sought out Dr. Weathers in San Bernardino and saw before me a stocky man with closely cropped hair and the look of a tough (but kindly) Marine Corps drill sergeant who has allowed middle age to turn muscle into the first signs of fat. After a quick tour of the ward where his patients are housed and a brief chat with a young man who was brought in after he had been found wandering in nearby mountains wearing nothing but a mystical trance, we drive to Dr. Weathers's ranch-style home in a modest neighborhood for lunch.

Over simple, but hearty, fare of soup and salad (all made from fresh ingredients) Weathers talks about vitamins, his wife nodding quiet assent. As he talks, his three-year-old son comes bouncing into the room. Weathers looks at the boy fondly. "He was born with holes in his heart and aortic stenosis [a condition in which a heart valve is too stiff to allow proper blood flow from the heart to the aorta]," Weathers says as the boy makes for his mother. "The doctors didn't think he would live. I gave him 400 international units of vitamin E every day. The last checkup showed that the holes in his heart had healed and the pressures inside the heart caused by the stenosis were back to normal."

The talk switches to his patients back at the hospital, one woman in particular. Weathers grimaces in disgust. "I'm just going to have to do something to get her out of that house she is living in," he says heatedly. "This woman has hypoglycemia and is schizophrenic. Yet her kindly old aunts insist on stuffing her with things like freshly baked apple pies, just exactly the kind of thing that she doesn't need." Every time this woman comes under his care, Weathers says, he gets her off her detrimental diet, watches her blood-sugar levels change, puts her on vitamins, and succeeds in stilling her emotional upheavals. But every time the woman goes home to her relatives, she relapses into her schizophrenic state.

Weathers shakes his head as he takes some soup. He brightens as an idea comes to him. "That's the exciting thing about biological psychiatry," he says (he prefers biological psychiatry as a term to orthomolecular psychiatry). "You can use laboratory methods like tests for hypoglycemia to a great extent to see and prove what you are doing. Psychiatry has always been a vague and esoteric art. Using some of these other techniques, it makes it much more of a practice of medicine."

By the time the mid-1970s had rolled around, Weathers had treated about five thousand patients with megavitamins. "I am not saying that all of them significantly improved in three months and are now working in good jobs," he told me at the time we talked. "But they are managing and functioning for the first time in a long time. It is really impressive to see someone who has been sitting around in the back room of the house for five years eating potato chips and watching television, taking high doses of tranquilizers—to see this individual respond and become more functional."

The widening enthusiasm for the orthomolecular approach to schizophrenia even spread—though temporarily—to at least one union, Los Angeles Retail Clerks Union, Local 770, a 25,000-member organization. The union's long-time president, Joe De-Silva, would fit almost anyone's stereotype image of an old-fashioned union leader. He is a small man who wears well-tailored suits but still moves with the awkward gait of a man who spent too much time doing too much heavy work, a man who has grown too accustomed to bending his knees and spreading his legs to lift and carry heavy packages.

For years DeSilva has been fascinated by mental illness and psychiatry. As far back as 1959 DeSilva negotiated a contract that included psychiatric coverage for his workers. But a few years ago, as the 1960s were drawing to a close, DeSilva grew disenchanted with traditional psychiatry and began to seek new treatments for mental illness—and for good reason. A close relative of his developed what he says was schizophrenia.

"She was in a mental hospital seven times," DeSilva says. "They told us to prepare ourselves for her permanent hospitalization. Then I found a book called *Biochemistry of Mental Disorders* and found that as far back as 1922 mental patients in the South were given niacin and that within one year they cleared 100,000 cases out of the psychotic wards.

"I decided that it might help, but first I began to take it myself because I wanted to see if the vitamin could cause injury. It made me feel good, so I gave it to her. Within three weeks she was a different person. She is now taking three grams of niacin a day and is perfectly normal. Sure, she still gets depressed sometimes, but now she can cope with it or call me on the phone and we talk about it until she feels better."

Struck by the apparent good effect the vitamin had on his loved one, DeSilva immersed himself in the megavitamin field, even organizing a symposium where various experts on schizophrenia could discuss this new therapy. ("I went because I got suckered into it," says one schizophrenia researcher who claims he had no advance knowledge that the symposium would be centered about nicotinic acid and orthomolecular psychiatry. "My God, it was like a political rally!") DeSilva set up an extensive library about mental illness. He made it possible for a chapter of Schizophrenics Anonymous to meet regularly in the building where the union was housed. Space in the union's medical benefits department was set aside for megavitamin literature, which was sold or given away to members of the union and outsiders seeking advice about emotional problems. In the department there were also shelvesful of megavitamins, which were sold to those union members who wanted to take them just to attain an improvement in their everyday physical and mental health, or to those who had consulted orthomolecular psychiatrists—from a list supplied by the union—for more serious emotional problems and who had been prescribed a megavitamin regimen.[1]

DeSilva was ultimately ousted from the presidency and retired from the union as well. His leadership of the union had come under attack for a number of reasons, but his messianic dedication to the megavitamin cause did nothing to help his position. After he left, megavitamins and megavitamin therapy advice were no longer dispensed from the union's headquarters. But after leaving the union, DeSilva formed an independent orthomolecular psychiatry information center in Hollywood.

The enthusiasm for megavitamins, for a time, even spread to the corridors of government. In the mid-1970s California State Senator James Mills heard a luncheon speech by Dr. Hoffer. Impressed by what he had heard, he discussed the Canadian's ideas with one of his aides—who mentioned that his brother was a schizophrenic. Concerned, Mills asked the aide what he thought could be done to help the brother. Simple, the aide answered, have the state's medical assistance program, Medi-Cal, pay for megavitamin therapy. Putting the controversial regimen under

---

[1] DeSilva was ultimately ousted from the presidency and retired from the union as well. His leadership of the union had come under attack, anyway, but his messianistic dedication to the megavitamin cause did nothing to help his position. After leaving the union, DeSilva formed an independent orthomolecular psychiatry information center in Hollywood.

state-supported medical coverage, the aide said, would help put it within the financial reach of mentally disturbed people who would not be able to afford it otherwise.

As a result of this conversation, Mills introduced several bills in the California legislature. One would have required Medi-Cal to pay for orthomolecular treatment, one would have authorized hospitals to conduct trials with megavitamins, another one would have ordered private medical insurance plans to cover megavitamin therapy, and, finally, one would have sanctioned controlled experiments with megavitamins at the Linus Pauling Institute of Science and Medicine. None of the bills saw the light of day. Two were dropped before the legislature had an opportunity to vote on them. Two were vetoed by then Governor Jerry Brown.

Undaunted, Mills tried again and in 1976 managed to gain approval of a bill that established demonstration projects in three California counties. As originally envisioned by Mills, the project would have assessed the medical and financial benefits of megavitamin therapy. But after a lot of bureaucratic and political haggling—the Department of Health Services didn't want to be responsible for evaluating the medical benefits of megavitamins and suggested the Department of Mental Health undertake the effort, a suggestion unacceptable to Mills—it was decided that the demonstration project would only be used to determine the financial impact of megavitamin therapy on the state's finances. The project finally got going and in April of 1979 was put in motion in Alameda, Orange, and Santa Cruz counties.

The study ran for fifteen months, until June of 1980. And, when it was over, the Department of Health Services could only conclude that "there were no significant increases or decreases in Medi-Cal costs when orthomolecular services were added." Largely because the demonstration project seemed to indicate that an orthomolecular project wouldn't make much difference to the state's treasury if it were to be included in Medi-Cal, megavitamin proponents managed to get another bill introduced which would have made the therapy a permanent part of the Medi-Cal reimbursment schedule. But opposition, particularly from the California Medical Association, doomed the bill and it died in committee.

The growing respectability of orthomolecular psychiatry—growing in the sense that more and more psychiatrists were willing to use it and that clinics like the San Bernardino Mental Health Unit and the North Nassau Mental Health Center had embraced it avidly—made it possible for disturbed men and women, as well as parents of disturbed children, to turn to orthomolecular psychiatrists without feeling pangs of doubt, without feeling that they were dealing with some arcane pseudo-science. That many people with the title "Doctor" or "Professor" before their name were endorsing megavitamin therapy gave thousands hope that previously uncontrollable and painful mental upheavals might at last be left beind.

As far as a woman named Ruby is concerned, megavitamins have ended her precipitous slide into an inevitable and permanent insanity. Ruby's husband, Barry, had been offered a job up in Toronto, Canada. Even though Ruby, a nervous and highly insecure woman, shook with fear about having to cope with so strange and unfamiliar an environment, they made the long move north.

Soon after their arrival in Toronto, her marriage started breaking up. The same emotions, insecurities that had kept her shy, lonely, essentially friendless throughout her life, were cropping up again, estranging her from her husband, making it increasingly impossible for her to deal with her marriage. "I thought I would try a psychiatrist to see if that would help," she says, talking in a depressed, almost monotonous voice. "But he wouldn't even give me any medication, not even sleeping pills I needed and begged him for. He was a very cruel man."

Within two years, Ruby found herself divorced from her husband. She had a breakdown and had herself institutionalized in a psychiatric hospital. "The only thing they did for me was put me on tranquilizers," she says, a touch of anger cutting occasionally through the monotone. "I didn't even get individual therapy because the psychiatrist in charge of me wanted me to participate in group sessions only. He refused to see me privately and I refused to go to the group sessions. I couldn't talk there. So I sat around, doing manual therapy like everybody else, knitting, pasting little tiles on boards, coloring pictures, or building boxes out of popsicle sticks. And listening to people talk about their latest suicide attempt. I checked out of that place, against my doctor's advice."

Ruby moved on to Los Angeles to live with her sister. Still determined to help herself, she found a chapter of the American Schizophrenia Association—a group formed by people associated with megavitamin therapy—and asked them to recommend a psychiatrist she could consult. "The doctors in Toronto told me that I was schizophrenic," Ruby explains. "And whenever I could get myself to read about it—reading about mental illness always scared me so much—all the symptoms seemed to fit my personality. So I had no doubts I was schizophrenic and called the Schizophrenia Association."

The doctor recommended to her, Dr. Harvey Ross, tested her for hypoglycemia, placed her on a sugar-free diet when the test results proved positive, and recommended a megavitamin regimen for her: nicotinamide, 3 grams a day; B complex, 50 milligrams a day; vitamin E, 1,200 international units a day; pyridoxine, 300 milligrams a day; ascorbic acid, 3 grams a day. The therapy, Ruby says, has helped.

"On the whole, I feel like a normal person for the first time in my life. Now I can read about mental illness and not get scared. I'm not depressed anymore, and for the first time in my life I feel really happy," she says.

"I did finally get my master's, but I still work as a secretary because I have trouble with my interviews. I still get frightened and shy and my mind goes blank and I don't paint as rosy a picture as I should of myself. I feel lonely and want to date because I would like to get married again. I have been answering those ads in the *Singles Register* [a Los Angeles tabloid newspaper for single people], but I haven't gotten any answers." She stops a moment, perhaps realizing that she is feeling sorry for herself. She cheers up. "But I joined two of those computer clubs and I am happily anticipating meeting people there."

Megavitamin patients who have relapsed into mental illness after stopping their megavitamin treatment are among the most ardent supporters of the orthomolecular approach. In his sixteenth year, Mrs. Cissy Landon says, her son Gary had suddenly begun to act strange, growing uncommunicative, irritable, and confused. His high grades, which had been B's and A's, suddenly deteriorated into C's and D's. Worried, Mrs. Landon took Gary to see two psychiatrists. Both told her her son was schizophrenic and should be hospitalized.

Unable to find an institution satisfactory to them, the Landons cast about for other alternatives. In time they heard about Dr. Hoffer's work. They contacted him, seeking his advice. He recommended they find a psychiatrist who used megavitamin therapy to treat schizophrenics. But at the time that Gary was sinking deeper and deeper into his insanity, no psychiatrist the Landons could find would consider the orthomolecular approach. "We decided to go on our own and administer the niacin according to the recommended dosage," Mrs. Landon says. "In August, 1965, our son began the niacin treatment—3,000 milligrams per day in doses of 500-milligram tablets three times a day, plus 1,000 milligrams of vitamin C. The change was obvious within a few weeks. He began functioning again as a human being, slowly emerging from the cocoon of silence and withdrawal in which he had wrapped himself. His school grades shot up amazingly. He was on no other medication. He was never on tranquilizers at any time. In fact, he was very much against taking pills of any kind and didn't even like taking the niacin, so it was not a matter of 'faith' on his part. To start out with, he indicated it wouldn't help."

One year after he had started on the megavitamin therapy and after starting classes in college, Gary stopped taking the niacin and the ascorbic acid. According to Mrs. Landon, Gary slipped back into some of the behavior patterns he had exhibited when he had been ill in high school.

"By the time our son had been off the niacin three and a half years," Mrs. Landon remembers, "the depression, extreme fatigue, irritability, mental confusion had come back. At this point he returned home and announced he would go back on the niacin. He also went on a low-blood-sugar diet. Again he responded in a completely positive way to this therapy." For the first time in his life, Gary, at the age of twenty-two, began to learn how to drive a car. He passed his licensing test, found a job working for a landscape architect and began to date. "He now has a girl friend for the first time in his life," Mrs. Landon adds. "We have seen enormous growth in this young man!"

As excitement over the use of vitamins in treating adult schizophrenics grew, it was inevitable that parents and doctors trying to cope with children stricken by an assortment of emotional and mental problems—childhood schizophrenia, autism, hyperactivity, an assortment of brain dysfunctions, learning disabilities—would also try the orthomolecular approach on their charges.

Among those who enthusiastically adopted megavitamins in the hope they would help children was Bernard Rimland, a San Diego psychologist—real title: senior scientist, Navy Personnel Research and Development Center—who has made a virtual second career, although a nonprofitable one, out of running the Institute for Child Behavior Research, a sort of clearinghouse for information and research about the learning, emotional, and psychiatric problems that afflict many children.

When I located the Institute for Child Behavior Research, it was crammed into the back room of Rimland's modest home in a middle-class San Diego neighborhood. Among the mountains of books and reports, among the cabinets that no longer had enough space for the constantly accumulating files, the letters and the case studies, Rimland had managed to isolate a niche for a desk and a couple of chairs. One of his assistants is busy catching up on paperwork in the crowded "office," so Rimland invites me out to the living room. Not that there is really a dividing line between home and institute. Journals on autistic children, on children with learning disabilities, on schizophrenic children, on hyperactive children spill out of the small back-room office into a hallway that links it to the dining room, into the dining room itself, and even into the adjacent living room.

Through his institute and through the National Association of Autistic Children, Rimland says, he constantly heard from parents about the latest therapies being advocated for disturbed children. There were therapies involving computers, music, shadow plays, complete deprivation of sight and sound, treatments that included LSD and other hallucinogenic drugs, treatments that included colonic purges. Every treatment, Dr. Rimland says, was hailed as a breakthrough. "At one point, I put vitamins in the same bag as the other fads," Rimland says. But then, he adds, he began to wonder, mainly because parents in widely divergent places—California, New York, Massachusetts, Georgia, even Europe—began writing him, telling him of the success they were having with vitamins. And all of them were saying the same thing: nicotinic acid, ascorbic acid, pyridoxine, pantothenic acid were doing wonders for their children. According to Rimland, he was "struck with the extent to which the trial-and-error efforts so often converged to the same group of three or four vitamins—the same vitamins, by and large, that biochemical research studies have implicated as perhaps being of the greatest relevance in mental disorders: niacin, ascorbic acid, pyridoxine, and, to a lesser degree, pantothenic acid. Well over half of the children for whom we received reports received significant improvement, irrespective of diagnosis, and children given various combinations of these four vitamins in particular often showed remarkable improvement."

Impressed by the spontaneous reports that were coming in to the institute, Rimland began to actively seek out parents (and physicians sympathetic to megavitamins) who had treated children with high vitamin dosages. "I have about ten children on the vitamins now," one psychiatrist wrote him. "Some of the results have been absolutely fantastic. At least half of the total 15 to 20 children whom I have placed on the vitamins have shown dramatic improvement." The mother of a nine-year-old boy who was placed on four grams of niacin, three grams of ascorbic acid, pyridoxine, and minerals, as well as other vitamins, wrote Rimland that the changes in her son were unbelievable. The boy, she said, was now "very sociable, more alert, more responsive." A Wisconsin mother gave her five-and-a-half-year-old son megavitamins because he was so hard to control in school. "Within a week after starting vitamins his behavior at nursery school began to improve," she wrote. "He began to follow orders, became less negative, and began to enjoy himself." A Canadian woman (whose own mother worked in one of the hospitals where Dr. Hoffer works and who sought him out for assurance that the vitamins would not be harmful to a youngster) told Rimland that when she put her badly behaved two-and-a-half-year-old son on vitamin C and nicotinamide, the improvement could be seen virtually overnight. "He appears normal to people," the mother reported. "They remark on his slowness of speech but otherwise make no allowance for his illness. Relatives and friends expect him to behave well, to listen to their orders, and correct him if he doesn't. This surprises me, since for such a long period no one cared what he did as long as he wasn't screaming."

Although megavitamins in the treatment of childhood emotional and neurological problems were first adopted and popularized by parents and a handful of interested professionals like Rimland, vitamin therapy for children came to find a more generalized acceptance, especially because more and more psychiatrists and doctors began to accept the argument that many of the disorders they were seeing in children have, like similar problems in adults, biochemical, not psychological, roots. The New York Institute for Child Development, an institution that specializes in treating severely disturbed children, was among the first child treatment centers to incorporate vitamins and special diets into their therapeutic programs. I visited the institute on a Wednesday, the day the NYICD's doctor is there to see children. The waiting room is busy, filled with anxious parents and their children. One couple has been there close to four hours, waiting to see the doctor. Another couple sit closely together, a look of dull resignation masking their faces. The woman holds a tiny girl in her lap. The child, head covered with blond curly hair, hangs limply, like a Raggedy Ann doll, in her mother's arms. She looks uncomprehendingly around the room, occasionally letting out a small birdlike trill. Faced by the crush of people outside, Dr. Alan Levin, the pediatrician who comes here on Wednesdays, has little time to see me. Between bites from a roast-beef sandwich brought in by a secretary, he tells me quickly why he uses vitamins on these children. "In my own practice I have seen a lot of these children and I had always wondered what to do with their behavioral and learning problems," Levin says, bolting down the sandwich in response to his assistant's frequent and nervous reminders that there are still people waiting to be seen. "All I was able to do was refer them to someone for remedial tutoring, but I began to feel that there had to be some biochemical insufficiency, some kind of an abnormality or deviation from normal that had to be changed to get an individual to function normally." Levin finishes his sandwich, gulps down the last of the coffee, and wipes his hands and mouth quickly with a paper napkin. His face is impatient, he wants to think of something to put across the point fast. "It's like taking an automobile that requires a premium gas and putting regular gas in the tank and finding that it will run, but run raggedly," he says in a rush as the assistant stomps in with a folder and casts him an angry look. "The human machine will run, but it won't run as well as it should in kids who need the megavitamins."

A number of private schools that specialize in educating emotionally disturbed children and children with learning disabilities have also adopted megavitamin therapy. One of the more prominent to do so at the height of the enthusiasm for megavitamins was the Churchill School in New York City, named after the British prime minister, who had his own early childhood educational problems. At three o'clock in the afternoon, the elegant old brownstone in which the school is located on Manhattan's fashionable Upper East Side shakes with the bedlam only children being released from a day of classes can create. They spill down the stairs in a cacophony of noise over assignments, lost gloves, and debates over rides home. At the school (founded by a New York socialite, Harry S. Valentine III, a serious but low-keyed young man) the children are treated with visual therapy, sensorimotor therapy (to sharpen their coordination), special tutoring. But their parents are encouraged to place their sons and daughters on high protein, low-carbohydrate diets, supplemented by megavitamins.

"We don't make the megavitamin therapy mandatory," Valentine, who also founded the New York Institute for Child Development, told me. "But from our experience at the institute we felt that hypoglycemic diets and vitamins could help children. When we administered doses of vitamins to hyperactive children and put them on a high-protein diet, we would often hear from the parents or from the teachers of startling changes in the children. They would say, 'We don't know what's come over Johnny! He is so well-behaved.'

"As a result of our experience at the institute, if a child here at the school exhibits symptoms such as hyperactivity or a short attention span or some borderline schizophrenic symptoms, we suggest to the parents that they look into the vitamin approach, although they are free to use conventional drugs if they want. About a third of our students are able to stick to the diet and the vitamins and I think they benefit from them."

Parents, educators, and professionals who have embraced megavitamins feel that they are effective because children given the vitamins show improvement they did not exhibit when treated with other drugs. One of them was Dr. Allan Cott, a New York psychiatrist who, when I talked to him, was one of the most fervent advocates of megavitamins. Megavitamins, he told me, have outperformed every other kind of therapy in alleviating the problems of the hundreds of children he treated with the regimen. "The children I have seen have been exposed to every form of treatment and every known tranquilizer and sedative with little or no success in controlling the hyperactivity," Dr. Cott says. On the megavitamins, he adds, "the children who are nonverbal begin to make definite vocal efforts. Many children report that the child begins to babble and become 'noisy.' Children who are already verbal make greater efforts to communicate through speech and often will begin to use phrases and short sentences to express wants and observations. They show a slow but steady improvement in speech. . . . They become more loving and not only permit cuddling and hugging but seek it. Bizarre food choices change slowly to include a larger variety of foods."

In general, Dr. Cott says, his experiences with megavitamin therapy have been nothing but successful. "In brain-injured children," he reports, "convulsions respond to megavitamin treatment. The parents of one patient reported that eleven days after starting their brain-injured child of [*sic*] vitamin B$_6$ he had his first seizure-free day in three years. During those three years he was taking Dilantin and phenobarbital daily and the seizure activity was not controlled." Still another patient who had had multiple seizures for two years, Dr. Cott says, was relieved within seventy-two hours after megavitamin therapy was begun, and has stayed seizure-free for almost four years. Summarizes Dr. Cott: "I have seen very few cases of childhood schizophrenia, autism, or brain injury in whom seizure activity did not respond to megavitamins."

The best proof that megavitamins work in children with assorted neurological and psychological problems, Dr. Rimland says, can be found in those children who, for one reason or another, have been taken off megavitamins briefly during the course of their struggles. One psychiatrist, Rimland says, tried megavitamins on a ten-year-old boy who was so violent and uncontrollable that he had to be hospitalized. The psychiatrist was not particularly sold on megavitamins, but since the desperate mother kept insisting they be tried, he at last relented. "To the surprise of [the doctor] and the delight of the mother and the nursing staff," Dr. Rimland says, "the boy's behavior showed marked improvement." The doctor,

Rimland goes on, was still skeptical, but decided to try the regimen on a thirteen-year-old boy who had been diagnosed as schizophrenic. "Again," Dr. Rimland says, "the results were excellent—for a short time. Dr. B., [Dr. Rimland identifies the physician only with an initial] puzzled, made an intensive study of everything he could think of which might have caused the relapse. On a hunch, he asked the hospital pharmacist for his prescription and found the answer. When the boy's first order of 500-milligram niacinamide tablets had been used up, the pharmacist had refilled the prescription with 50-milligram tablets because the second 'o' in '500' was not clear. On the higher dosage again, the patient's behavior began to improve." A mother who had reduced her child's intake of pantothenic acid wrote Dr. Rimland that when the dosage was lowered from 900 milligrams to 300 milligrams a day, "I at first noticed no change, but after one and a half months, it suddenly hit me that he was listless again. He was sucking his thumb, not running about, irritable . . . spontaneity was gone. Up went the pantothenic acid and the spontaneity returned immediately. I'll never do that again."

Like their counterparts who deal with adult schizophrenics, those who favor the use of megavitamins as a treatment therapy for autistic, schizophrenic, and learning-disabled children are resigned to being unable to convince the bulk of the conventional psychiatrists and educators that vitamins do make a difference. "The people who are threatened by it," says Harry Valentine, "are the professors who have written books about how to deal with learning disabilities. They think it is nonsense and give you a hard time. But a person on the firing line who has to cope with kids will try anything that will help."

Many professionals, says Rimland, just won't believe the effectiveness of the megavitamins even when they come face to face with their results. "We know of a kid in Utah," Rimland recalls, slouching down into the living-room couch, throwing one arm over his head, "who had improved on vitamins. The psychiatrist said it was due to his therapy, not the vitamin 'nonsense.' The mother took him off the vitamins for a month and the kid cried and screamed. The mother said, see, I took him off the vitamins. Everybody laughed. But the psychiatrist couldn't do a thing with him and on one of the visits to the doctor's office, she couldn't even get him out of the car, the doctor had to come out of his office to see him. 'He's regressed,' he told her. She took him home, gave him the vitamins, and he got better in half an hour.''

''Individual doctors won't accept proof, even if they see it with their own eyes, until some official body tells them it is okay to believe,'' Dr. Cott says, talking at the same time that he is busily doing his paper work at the end of a busy day. ''One of the first children I treated was a psychotic child, schizophrenic, completely disturbed. He had been in the children's division of a mental hospital because he could not be controlled at home. He was the sickest, most psychotic thing I have ever seen. Fortunately he was one of the kids who get dramatic improvement on vitamins. After two years the mother was so proud that she made an appointment with the psychiatrist who had made the original diagnosis and had told her to put the kid away because nothing was going to help him. The doctor looked at this kid. He pulled out his folder. He looked at Jackie again, who was sitting there behaving himself like a nice little kid, and the doctor's comment was, 'This can't be right, I must have made a mistake in the diagnosis.' He retracted his diagnosis rather than believe what he saw. In his experience he had never seen a schizophrenic child improve in this way in that short a time.''

There is, it is true, widespread skepticism about the effectiveness of vitamins in children with behavioral and educational problems. One southern California doctor, Robert D. Carpenter, a general practitioner who specializes in treating hyperactive children, says that at first he was impressed by the reports on megavitamins and was eager to try them in his practice. The results, he says, were disappointing. "I tried them on thirty different children," Dr. Carpenter says. "Now, in one case the results were very dramatic. It was a kindergarten student who had been causing so much trouble that he was on the verge of being expelled. The mother gave the boy Ritalin, Dilantin, Mellaril. They helped, but not very much. I told the mother about megavitamins, that I had just heard about them and she said, at this point I'll try anything. I gave her the information. Within a month's time, he had had a dramatic improvement. We stopped the Ritalin and he has continued doing quite well."

"I got one or two other children in which they seemingly had some benefit. The other twenty-five children, however, did not respond at all. If what Cott says is true, I would have hoped for at least fifty-fifty results with the megavitamins. What I got were some pretty slim pickings."

Researchers at a mental hospital in Camarillo, California, also tried to replicate Dr. Cott's positive megavitamin results. "There were some changes in the children who received them, but nothing convincing," says Mrs. Carolyn B. Downs, a Los Angeles educator who works with disturbed children and who observed the study. "One child who had not said the word 'purple' in two years said it. A child who had been self-destructive stopped being so. Other children were throwing fewer tantrums and were more open to suggestion. The results started showing in six weeks and everybody got very excited. But then the positive signs started to fade away. I'm not convinced that the initial improvements were not because the children got more attention during the course of the study and because perhaps more was expected of them."

(Other people who have dealt extensively with children who suffer from various dysfunctions also tend to agree that the changes observed sometimes after megavitamins are administered come about, not as a function of the vitamins, but as a function of the changed expectations of those who deal with the children. "As far as many parents are concerned," says Mrs. Lillian Seymour, a past officer of the California Association for Neurologically Handicapped Children, a woman who had learning problems in her own childhood and who has a brain-damaged son, "the effectiveness of megavitamins might just be a self-fulfilling prophecy. If a doctor tells a parent that the child is getting better, and if the parents are paying a lot of money for the treatment and the vitamins, that can subtly change their own attitudes toward the child. They start easing up on the pressure—at the dinner table, about performance in school—and in taking the pressure off, the child often changes for the better. When you send some of these children to a therapeutic camp where there are no pressures and the director and the counselors work to create situations in which the child will succeed, the hyperactivity often decreases. Take this kid out of camp, send him back to regular school and its pressures, and the emotional disturbance returns.")

Many experts also tend to be skeptical about megavitamins because there have been no rigorous double-blind studies performed with megavitamin therapy on disturbed children, because megavitamin therapists intertwine some very conventional drugs with their vitamin regimens. Dr. Cott, Dr. Carpenter says, tailors his approach to megavitamin therapy to suit his audience. "In an article in *Prevention* [a magazine for vitamin and health-food enthusiasts]," Dr. Carpenter says, "he mentions only megavitamins and Mellaril. When he wrote me when I asked for advice on how to use vitamins, he mentioned a much broader scope of traditional medicine, including Ritalin."

Dr. Cott shrugs off the criticism but is hard pressed to control rising anger over the remark that others demand double-blind studies and mention of the criticism that he and other megavitamin therapists use a gunshot approach to megavitamin therapy, that they don't really know what is helping the child. "I sure as hell wouldn't want to have one of my kids be part of a double-blind study," he says, glaring over the half-frame reading glasses he wears down toward the end of his nose. "Why should the child be denied real treatment just to be made part of an experiment? If a controlled study runs over a two-year period and the child during this time is on a placebo at various intervals, that's a criminal thing to do. You are denying that child treatment at a very critical year in its life. One doesn't have a lot of years with a learning-disabled child, because if he doesn't make it by the age of about twelve, his academic career is gone.

"I don't give a damn what's helping the child, all I am interested in is that I am helping him. Certainly I would like to have it pinpointed so he doesn't have to take so many things. Until we know exactly what is doing what, we don't know which vitamins to give and which ones to leave out. So therefore we have to go along doing the best we can on an empirical basis."

It is hard, however, to accept an argument for megavitamins (as it is hard to accept an argument for any kind of new, theoretical medical treatment) on purely empirical grounds. To do so would be to accept, with really not much proof, the word of people who are not in a position to judge results objectively—no matter how much they protest that they can be fair-minded. Any doctor who advocates a new form of therapy has to see it in a positive light because he has a double-vested interest in it. He quite obviously has a financial reason to hope that his new regimen will work. That will bring him an increasing number of new patients. And he has an egotistical reason as well to hope that his ideas are accepted: that would make him famous and acclaimed.

Moreover, it is hard to accept much of the so-called empirical proof for megavitamin therapy because much of it comes from people who have even less capacity for objective judgment than the physicians who practice with vitamins: it comes from people, after all, who have good reason to wish, ardently, that what they are now taking or giving their children will prove to be more effective than the last drug in alleviating either their own miseries or those of their children.

To base a whole new medical approach on the testimony of parents who have children they have not been able to handle, it seems, is especially risky. One has to wonder, for example, how many parents of disturbed or brain-damaged children report that their children are getting better on megavitamins because they have to believe that the child is improving. Many parents who have disturbed children suffer from soul-racking guilt feelings. Somehow they believe that they are responsible for their child's misfortune, that they have done something terribly wrong that has somehow resulted in this awful curse on an innocent life. To give a child megavitamins, which ostensibly correct a theoretical biochemical malfunction, is to correct a purely physiological accident that has nothing really to do with their worthiness as parents. In an article Dr. Cott illustrates the point well (though unwittingly): "Since most parents who have sought professional help have been exposed to the psychodynamic orientation, they have been given an added burden of guilt by being blamed for the child's illness. Clarification of the condition helps the parents to realize that they are not to blame and enables them to manage the child with greater consistency and less over-protectiveness. With the understanding of the biochemical nature of the disorder, parents are given hope of improvement in their child's condition by the use of chemotherapy." Or, as Dr. Rimland told one group of parents of autistic children: "I think that you will agree with me that we are on the right track, for at least a good number of our children. While we are still a long way from having all the answers, we have accomplished an important first step. As our analyses and studies continue we will develop a great deal of further, needed information. This approach seems a lot more productive than the old one of 'Blaming the Parents,' doesn't it?''

Empirical proof for a regimen coming from parents who have a deep need for that proof just does not count as truth in the search for scientific validity. Never mind parents who cannot convince themselves, without giving their children massive doses of vitamins, that they are not responsible for their child's misfortunes. One has to wonder how many parents, exasperated by a rambunctious child, an overactive child, decide, largely by themselves, that the child is seriously and profoundly disturbed and needs medical help—help they proceed to administer by themselves in the form of megavitamin treatment for several months or even years. If in that time the child changes for the better, who is to say that the simple act of growing up might not have changed the child anyway? Can one embrace megavitamins, can one prescribe them on a ''empirical'' basis because some woman in Canada—a woman we know nothing about, whose tolerance for her child is a mystery to us—writes to say that it was the vitamins that caused her son to change over a period of two and a half years when he would have undergone maturational changes anyway?

We can't, rather, shouldn't take this kind of testimonial to heart. Certainly the medical profession, which has to be accountable for what it pours into people, ought not to take this kind of evidence as proof positive. Vitamins, in massive doses, are not the innocuous substances we would like them to be. In massive doses, they are drugs. And if they are drugs, we should demand that they be tested in the same rigorous fashion in which other pharmaceutical substances are tested. Since the megavitamin therapists have refused to carry out the kind of studies the medical and scientific community demand, it is small wonder that so-called establishment researchers felt compelled to undertake the studies and even smaller wonder that they could not, after studying the results they had garnered, voice the same sanguine hopes for megavitamin therapy.

CHAPTER VI

Counterattack

For as long as they could, the medical and scientific communities studiously ignored orthomolecular psychiatry. As the movement gained momentum, however, it became increasingly difficult to dismiss its pressures with a shrug of indifference. Newspapers and magazines, drawn by the shimmering promises of the new specialty, opened their pages to the advocates of megavitamin therapy. Emotionally ill men and women who read these articles, and who had heard that this friend or that acquaintance had seemingly made startling progress under the guidance of an orthomolecular psychiatrist, were seeking out these new practitioners or were confronting their own psychiatrists, demanding nicotinic acid and other vitamins, asking for a hypoglycemic diet. Almost every time a schizoprenia researcher or a psychiatrist opened up a professional journal—whether it was the *Journal of Nervous and Mental Diseases,* the *Canadian Medical Association Journal, Psychosomatics,* whatever—there was another orthomolecular psychiatrist describing his latest series of nicotinic acid triumphs in a long article or arguing the vitamin's merits in a letter to the editor. At conventions, meetings, and informal gatherings, there, unavoidably, was this new band of zealots touting its spectacular achievements in treating schizophrenics.

And so, when the counterattack got under way, fed by an impatience with the scientifically imprecise proofs presented by the orthomolecularists, it quickly built into a sometimes bitter, sometimes harsh, almost always uncompromising offensive. Orthomolecular psychiatrists, some critics began to say, had fallen for a sophomoric biochemical theory and had allowed themselves to be led off into an ill-advised scientific tangent, and were heading into a psychiatric cul-de-sac. Schizophrenia, these critics of orthomolecular psychiatry pointed out, is one of the most—if not the most—diabolically complicated of mental illnesses. And that even so scientifically sophisticated a figure as Linus Pauling could falter in the morass surrounding the illness, the critics said, was proof enough that *anyone* who professed to believe in nicotinic acid was also hopelessly confused. Dr. Pauling's 1968 dissertation on the orthomolecular origins of mental illness, Dr. Donald Oken, chairman of the Department of Psychiatry at the State University of New York at Syracuse, charged, "illustrates elegantly the pitfalls which occur when an expert in one field enters another area. With his characteristic brilliance, Linus Pauling describes a biochemical mechanism which could be responsible for some forms of mental illness. . . . Remote plausibility, however, no matter how intriguing and creative its nature, should not be confused with evidence. . . . While Pauling is widely knowledgeable and his chemistry may be impeccable, it is unfortunately evident that he is unfamiliar with the subtleties of methodology in a field in which he is untrained. Although this is understandable, it would be regrettable if the impact of his prestige and brilliance in other fields leads readers to believe otherwise and to accept unwisely what remains, on the basis of current knowledge, a wild speculation."

For other critics the theoretical and philosophical niceties of why the orthomolecular psychiatrists are wrong are not as important as the disturbing side effects—physiological and psychological—nicotinic acid could produce in some people. High doses of nicotinic acid, some doctors and psychiatrists have warned, can lead to nausea, vomiting, diarrhea, and flareups in peptic ulcers. Nicotinic acid can increase the levels of sugar in the blood, a dangerous problem for diabetics. In some cases, doctors warn, nicotinic acid, because it can dilate blood vessels all over the body at the same time, can cause a sudden and dangerous drop in blood pressure. Massive doses of the vitamin can cause chronic and disturbing flushing (because the vitamin dilates blood vessels, including those that supply the skin) and could also induce chronic itching in 30 to 60 percent of those taking the vitamin. Nicotinic acid can also darken the skin and make it rough, especially in the folds of the body. Although megavitamin therapists argue that these side effects are rare or can be mitigated with judicious use of other drugs or alternate forms of the vitamin (substituting nicotinamide, for example) the fact nevertheless remains, critics say, that the vitamin is not as innocuous as those who prescribe it want to believe. "The fact that most of these symptoms disappear upon discontinuance of NA [nicotinic acid] administration offers little support to the megavitamin therapy rationale, as its proponents consistently emphasize that many 'schizophrenics' may require extremely long-term periods of B_3 therapy—some, indeed, for life," a report by the American Psychiatric Association on orthomolecular psychiatry points out. "In view of the possible severely toxic consequences of sustained administration of megadoses of B_3, and in view of the paucity of present evidence indicating a conclusive answer either pro or contra on this question, it certainly cannot be responsibly maintained without qualification that B_3 in megadoses is a 'completely safe' pharmacological agent."

Some physicians worry that all the hip-hip-hoorah talk about nicotinic acid therapy and the relative simplicity of the regimen can mislead emotionally disturbed people into treatment shortcuts. "Uncritical acceptance of an unproven treatment," two New Haven, Connecticut, physicians, George R. Heninger and Malcolm Bowers, wrote the *Journal of the American Medical Association,* "generates a false sense of security which may delay or prevent proper medical treatment."

The two physicians reported that they had treated a twenty-five-year-old man who, since his graduation from college two years earlier, had been having increasingly frequent bouts of apathy and depression, coupled with feelings of loneliness and worthlessness. Concerned about his problems, and aware of some of the reports about the effectiveness of nicotinic acid, the man, during one of his fits of depression, took one and a half grams of nicotinic acid within an hour and a half. He apparently did not know that nicotinic acid could cause a flush and the characteristic heat of blood rushing through his dilated blood vessels frightened him. "Within a few hours," Heninger and Bowers reported, "the first of a series of uncontrollable crying spells occurred with continuous feelings of panic and the need for close physical contact. The following day the patient smoked marihuana [*sic*]. Whereas marihuana smoking had been pleasant on four previous occasions, this time he became terrified, felt that his mind was drifting away, and that he had lost his identity. In addition, the patient began to experience frightening dreams. These symptoms gradually increased in severity so that hospitalization was necessary five days later.''

Another of their patients, a twenty-eight-year-old unmarried writer, had taken three LSD trips. The first had been a fairly pleasant experience, but the other two had deteriorated into bad trips, one worse than the other. A psychiatrist, also a friend of the writer, suggested he take three grams of nicotinic acid a day to offset the aftereffects of the bad trips. After starting on the regimen, the writer took a fourth LSD trip, this time in the presence of his psychiatrist friend. Although the initial reaction to the LSD seemed favorable, Heninger and Bowers said, the writer began to have delusions, which grew increasingly bizarre. Four days later he had to be hospitalized. ''There is suggestive evidence,'' Doctors Heninger and Bowers wrote, ''that the pharmacologic effects of niacin (the flush in the case of the first patient, an amphetamine-like reaction in the case of the writer) potentiated the psychotic symptoms in the two cases. . . . In both cases, following niacin, drug experiences which had previously been mainly pleasant ones turned into frightening psychotic experiences.''

(Dr. Hoffer was, quite naturally, incensed at the Heninger-Bowers letter to *JAMA* and their ''sweeping claims based upon two cases in which treatment or self-treatment included a multitude of other variables such as LSD, hashish and curious forms of psychotherapy.'' It was impossible, Dr. Hoffer wrote in anger, to accept the theory that niacin would bring on psychotic incidents on the basis of experience with just two patients. ''Since 1952 I have treated over 1,000 patients with niacin and other chemotherapies using 3 to 30 grams per day,'' Dr. Hoffer retorted. ''I have seen none remotely resembling these cases reported. Many patients do not respond to niacin alone and in the natural history of their psychosis may be worse. One might as well explain a relapse in the evening as being due to a toxic reaction to the supper the patient had at 6 P.M. Since there are no chemicals [including water] wholly devoid of toxicity, it is not illogical for us to recommend as we always have done that vitamin B_3 therapy is best undertaken under a physician's care. I challenge any physician to provide evidence that niacin is as toxic as tranquilizers, anti-depressants, or any other chemotherapy used in psychiatry.''

Other psychiatrists, however, who practice with megavitamins do acknowledge a bit more readily that nicotinic acid can create panic states and might even activate a psychosis. But, these psychiatrists say, the side effects can be controlled. Says Dr. H. L. Newbold, an Ashville, North Carolina, psychiatrist: ''Those of us who administer niacin are well aware of this fact and know that if excitement appears, it can readily be held down, preferably by the use of diazepam [Valium]. I administer anywhere from 40 to 100 mg of diazepam daily and gradually decrease the level. With this technique the side effect can be rather easily managed.'')

Admittedly, Doctors Heninger and Bowers said, no hard-and-fast conclusions could be drawn from just two cases. Yet other researchers have also reported that nicotinic acid—perhaps because in vast doses it does sometimes act like amphetamine, causing high states of excitement—seems to worsen psychotic conditions in some mental patients. According to three researchers—Herbert Meltzer, Richard Shader, and Lester Grinspoon—a controlled study they had conducted with ten patients over a two-year period showed that patients treated with a nicotinic acid derivative and no tranquilizers exhibited tendencies ''toward increased hostility, aggressiveness and irritability beginning one week after initiation of . . . treatment and lasting for nearly two weeks after the [nicotinic acid derivative] was discontinued.''

The Meltzer article went further in giving nicotinic acid a negative assessment. The patients who were chosen for the study were ten men who had been diagnosed as chronic schizophrenics and who had been hospitalized for at least five years. In the two years before the experiment with nicotinic acid had begun, the men had shown distinct improvement in their conditions in response to other treatments, including tranquilizers and psychotherapy. If the megavitamin practitioners were correct, the Meltzer group suggested, these patients, whose disease had not reached the point of no return, should have reacted favorably and quickly to the trial doses of nicotinic acid they were given. None in fact did.

The Heninger-Bowers letter and the Meltzer article were only part of the critical counterattack now gathering force. Three researchers at the University of Western Ontario reported in the *Canadian Psychiatric Association Journal* that an experiment with fifty-four chronic schizophrenic patients from the Psychiatric Institute at Westminster Hospital in London, Ontario, had also failed to turn up any evidence that nicotinic acid was effective in treating schizophrenia.

A study conducted by Dr. J. Richard Wittenborn at Rutgers University also failed to confirm the claims made for megavitamin therapy. Eighty-six patients, fairly young and in early stages of their disease, were divided into two groups—one receiving nicotinic acid, the other a placebo—and followed for up to two years. Each group spent some time in the hospital. But all the patients, because psychiatrists believe that schizophrenics should spend as much time as possible in their homes and the community, spent a considerable amount of time away from the institution. Social workers visited the patients at home to interview them and their families. The patients visited the hospital's outpatient clinic once a month, where they were given physical examinations and were interviewed by a psychiatrist and a psychologist.

One of the claims made by the megavitamin therapists is that schizophrenic patients treated with nicotinic acid need rehospitalization less often than patients treated with other methods available. But, Dr. Wittenborn said, when the two groups in his study were compared, there was no difference in their rehospitalization rates. Forty-three percent of those who received the placebo over the course of the experiment had to be readmitted to the hospital. Forty-three percent of the group receiving nicotinic acid also had to be readmitted to the hospital. Over the entire period of the experiment, Dr. Wittenborn said, both the placebo patients and the nicotinic acid patients required fewer and fewer tranquilizers. At the end of the first month of the experiment, 87 percent of those in the nicotinic acid group required a major tranquilizer, whereas 96 percent of those receiving the placebo required something to quiet them down. However, at the end of the study, the number of patients in both groups requiring a major tranquilizer hovered at about 75 percent. "Careful comparative analysis of the data," Dr. Wittenborn concluded, "revealed very little difference between the responses of the two treatment groups and no definite indication of a therapeutic advantage for the supplemental use of niacin. Despite the reassuring clinical observation of Hoffer and others, the present findings challenge claims of general efficacy for a two-year regimen of niacin supplementation in the treatment of schizophrenia.''

Because of the growing clamor over nicotinic acid—a clamor by now being fed by those who were vigorously protesting the therapy as well as by those fighting harder to give it credibility—the Canadian Mental Health Association commissioned Dr. Thomas Ban to head a massive collaborative study into the effectiveness of megavitamin therapy. The choice, the CMHA felt, was eminently fair. Dr. Ban is an acknowledged psychiatric researcher. He had come from Hungary in 1956 and since his arrival in Canada had won two major prizes for psychiatric research. He is an associate professor of psychiatry and director of psychopharmacology at McGill University in Montreal, chief of research services at one hospital, and research consultant to three others. He and a collaborator, Dr. Heinz E. Lehmann, the man who introduced tranquilizers to North America, were considered to have a definite bias toward the belief that schizophrenia has a biochemical origin and that the disease can be treated biochemically. They were not prejudiced, in other words, by some blind faith in a Freudian explanation for the disease or by a preference for psychotherapeutic solutions to the problem.

Dr. Ban designed a study that ultimately was to coordinate twelve experiments, involving five hospitals and 360 patients. Every effort was made, the CMHA says, to take Dr. Hoffer's views and prescribed methods of treatment into consideration. Nevertheless, not one of the first four studies, carried out over a period of four years, confirmed the orthomolecularist faith in nicotinic acid.

One study, for example, included 30 patients whose disease had set in only shortly before the experiment had begun and who had been diagnosed as acute or subacute schizophrenics (in medicine, "acute" is, relatively speaking, good because it means that the disease may be severe but has not yet entrenched itself). The patients were divided into three groups, one group receiving nicotinic acid, one receiving nicotinamide, and one receiving a placebo. At the end of the study, Ban and his co-workers found that the patients receiving the nicotinic acid and the nicotinamide required a higher total amount and a higher average daily amount of tranquilizers than the group receiving only the placebo. Moreover, the placebo-group members spent less time in the hospital than those schizophrenics who had been assigned to the nicotinic acid or nicotinamide groups. "The most important single finding that emerged from this study was that no statistically significant difference in therapeutic action was evident in the three groups," Dr. Ban and his co-workers reported. "The addition of nicotinic acid or nicotinamide to the regular phenothiazine treatment regimen for a period of six months did not have any measurable therapeutic effect in these patients."

All in all, the Canadian Mental Health Association summarized, "findings in these studies strongly suggest that nicotinic acid therapy is not the optimal treatment for the average schizophrenic patient. . . . The overall therapeutic efficacy of nicotinic acid as the sole medication in newly admitted schizophrenic patients is not superior to the overall therapeutic efficacy of an inactive placebo. In fact the majority of newly admitted schizophrenic patients cannot be sufficiently controlled with high dosages of nicotinic acid administration. The overall efficacy of nicotinic acid as an adjuvant medication in newly admitted schizophrenic patients is inferior to the overall therapeutic efficacy of an inactive placebo. In fact the addition of nicotinic acid to regular phenothiazine treatment prolongs the duration of hospital stay. . . ."

The escalating "establishment" reaction to the growing influence of orthomolecular psychiatry in the lay population (and in some niches of the psychiatric community) led the American Psychiatric Association to appoint a special task force to look into the burgeoning phenomenon. The task force, headed by Dr. Morris Lipton, a psychiatrist and biochemist at the University of North Carolina Medical School, included, among others, Dr. Ban, Dr. Lehmann, and Dr. Wittenborn. No psychiatrists from the orthomolecular side were asked to participate. Rather than undertake a new, long, expensive study of its own, the task force reviewed the experiments conducted by the protagonists on both sides of the question and studied their reports in various journals. The result (perhaps not surprisingly, given the composition of the task force) was a blistering, no-holds-barred report that made short shrift of every orthomolecular claim made.

At the time the Lipton study was being conducted, many of the patients who were under orthomolecular therapy were also receiving ECT as well as powerful tranquilizers. Thus, the task force pointed out, the very title "orthomolecular" is a sham. "There is nothing orthomolecular," the report stated, "about the electroconvulsive therapy or the psychotropic drugs which hospitalized and many outpatients receive."

There was absolutely no convincing evidence in anything it had seen and read, the task force said, that backed up the claims made for orthomolecular psychiatry. "In our view the results and claims of the advocates of megavitamin therapy have not been confirmed by several groups of psychiatrists and psychologists experienced in psychopharmacological research," the report said. "The negative results have been obtained with adequately sized populations, employing standardized, reliable psychological and behavioral rating scales and appropriate statistics. . . . The claims the megavitamin proponents made as far back as 1957 have not been confirmed.

"We regret this conclusion because some good may have come out of this method of treatment. Guilt and shame have probably been reduced in both patients and their families because a metabolic disease is somehow easier to bear than a psychogenic illness. . . . Socially desirable outcomes have sometimes been derived from myths or fervently held beliefs. To this extent the orthomolecular movement in psychiatry may be socially useful. But if psychiatry is to become and remain scientific, it must meet the test of scientific validity. Nicotinic acid therapy does not do so at this time.

"In the end the credibility of the megavitamin proponents and the orthomolecular psychiatrists becomes the crucial issue because it is never possible to fully prove or disprove a therapeutic procedure. Rather the theory and practice gain or lose credibility as its premises, methods and results are examined, and attempts are made at clinical replication by independent investigators. This review and critique has carefully examined the literature produced by megavitamin proponents and by those who have attempted to replicate their basic and clinical work. It concludes that in this regard the credibility of the megavitamin proponents is low."

The orthomolecularists, of course, were not pleased with the findings of the Lipton group. Dr. Pauling, as their spokesman, complained in an article in the *American Journal of Psychiatry* that the Lipton task force's report was off base in many respects, including its failure to consider important evidence pointing a key role for ascorbic acid in schizophrenia and the task force's insistence on shunning evidence in favor of niacin. The task force report, Pauling wrote, did not discuss "the many papers in which a low level of ascorbic acid in the blood of schizophrenics is reported. Neither the general theory of orthomolecular psychiatry . . . nor any of the special arguments about the value of ascorbic acid is presented or discussed in any significant way . . . The evidence that niacin has no value is far from conclusive . . ."

Perhaps most important, Pauling took umbrage at the task force's insistence that the proponents of orthomolecular therapy had not sought to carry out well-designed, double-blind studies of their theories and that the vitamin enthusiasts, as a result, lacked credibility.

"I have talked with the leading orthomolecular psychiatrists and have found that they feel the principles of medical ethics prevent them from carrying out controlled clinical tests, with half of their patients receiving orthomolecular therapy in addition to the conventional treatment and the other half receiving only the conventional treatment," Pauling wrote. "It is the duty of the physician to give every one of his patients the treatment that in his best judgment will be of the greatest value. Some psychiatrists, including Hoffer and Osmond, carried out controlled trials 20 years ago. They became convinced that orthomolecular therapy, along with conventional treatment, was beneficial to almost every patient. From that time on their ethical principles have required that they give this treatment and not withhold it from half of their patients."

Pauling added: "The task force is wrong in criticizing the orthomolecular psychiatrists for not having carried out controlled clinical trials during the last few years. Instead, it is the critics, who doubt the value of orthomolecular methods, who are at fault in not having carried out well-designed clinical tests."

The findings by Ban, Lipton, and others that megavitamins are not all they are touted to be has, unfortunately, not diminished the fervor with which orthomolecular treatment is still greeted in many quarters. "None of these developments has dampened the enthusiasm of megavitamin practitioners," notes Dr. Barrett. "In fact while most of the controversy has centered about the treatment of schizophrenia, megavitamin proponents do not limit themselves to that condition. They are also treating mentally retarded children as well as adults with depression and various other emotional disorders—at fees which range as high as $500 for the initial psychiatric evaluation.''

That the orthomolecular psychiatrists and the "establishment" psychiatrists should come to such drastically differing positions on the value of nicotinic acid specifically, and the value of the entire orthomolecular regimen generally, in treating schizophrenia is hardly surprising. There is virtually nothing along the road to their separate conclusions that they do agree upon.

Dr. Hoffer and others complain bitterly that most studies conducted to test the orthomolecular claims are conducted only with nicotinic acid. The critics readily admit that they often limit the scope of their experiments. "We made a point of stressing that the only vitamin we thoroughly checked out was nicotinic acid," Dr. Lipton told me over the telephone. "But nicotinic acid is the cathedral of their ideology. If you can't believe the nicotinic acid, you can't believe the rest." In this respect, it must be said, the critics of orthomolecular psychiatry are right. Peter, Daniel, the seventy-three-year-old professor, P.F.—many of Hoffer's early cure claims—received no vitamin E, no hypoglycemic diets, no pyridoxine as adjuncts in their regimen, but nicotinic acid in huge doses. It is this vitamin and the vitamin alone that Hoffer and others credit for some of the astounding results obtained with the mentally ill.

Since Hoffer made his first claims, however, the nicotinic acid component of the therapy has come to be buried under layer after layer of additional ingredients. How is it possible, critical researchers ask, to make some sense out of a therapy when it is impossible to pinpoint which part of the therapy—including the therapy's cornerstone—is doing what? "When a serious attempt is made to replicate the clinical experiments under the specific conditions for which the original claims were made," the APA task force complains, "one finds that the conditions have changed. Orthomolecular psychiatrists constantly protest that failures to replicate their results stem from inappropriate selection of patients and from the failure to utilize all the components in their present program. The latter claim is probably correct because it is virtually impossible to replicate studies in which each patient receives a highly individualized therapeutic program with from one to seven vitamins in huge doses, plus hormones, special diets, other drugs and ECT, which are added or subtracted not on the basis of proven biochemical abnormalities but rather on the basis of the clinicians' individual judgment as to the patient's needs.'' Orthomolecular psychiatrists shrug off the criticism. He could do these studies to pinpoint just exactly what is in the megavitamin therapy that is working, Dr. Hawkins says. He could have taken the girl whose family had already spent a quarter of a million dollars on her and for the sake of scientific research have given her one ingredient at a time to see which would bring about the final cure. "But I couldn't do that," Dr. Hawkins says. "She ain't mice or rats, but a twenty-four-year-old girl with a life to live. I don't know why this girl is well on a scientific basis. I'm not interested really. I'm only interested in the fact that she is well."

Nor is there very much agreement on the question of diagnosis. Despite the great and obvious difficulties in identifying schizophrenia, megavitamin therapists, to the chagrin of other psychiatrists, insist on using a controversial biochemical test—the test for a pink spot or mauve factor in the urine—and an oversimplified true-false test to arrive at their decisions that patients are or are not schizophrenic. The mauve spot, Dr. Hoffer and others maintain, is caused by an abnormal biochemical process peculiar to schizophrenics. Other psychiatric researchers point out that the mauve spot appears in many other people as well. One researcher found it in twelve out of nineteen schizophrenics. But he also found it in thirteen out of nineteen garden-variety neurotics. Other researchers say they have found the mauve factor in at least one third of those patients with anxiety neurosis, alcoholism, mental retardation, depression, and personality problems.

The card-sorting test—called the Hoffer-Osmond Diagnostic or HOD test after its originators—is also highly suspect, psychiatrists experienced in diagnosis say. In the HOD test, the patient is asked to sort cards bearing 145 simple statements—"People's faces sometimes pulsate as I watch them," "My sense of hearing is now more sensitive than it ever has been," "At times my mind goes blank," "Praise is like punishment because they both start with a *p* rather than because they are given to people"—into true and false piles. The tester studies the way the cards have been assorted and then makes his diagnosis on that basis. According to Dr. Hoffer, the method is 90 percent accurate in diagnosing schizophrenia.

But, the APA committee says, the HOD test is open to several criticisms. Dr. Ban and Dr. Wittenborn have found that many acute and chronic schizophrenics are too ill to perform the test. The questions on the HOD test, the APA feels, are too ambiguous, too vague. Independent researchers who have tried to assess the test, the APA says, have come to contradictory conclusions. One researcher found that the HOD test could not distinguish between a simple neurotic and a schizophrenic. Other researchers found that the HOD could distinguish between schizophrenics, neurotics, and others with character disorders, but not between schizophrenics and other psychotics. All in all, the APA task force felt, "systematic scrutiny of the questions in the test by several experienced psychiatrists and psychologists yield the impression that it is far from specific for schizophrenia and that manics, depressives, and even anxiety neurotics might be diagnosed schizophrenic by this test."

The sharpest debates between orthomolecularists and other psychiatrists have erupted when experimental methodology is discussed, when researchers on both sides of the argument debate just how an experiment should be designed to determine whether or not the orthomolecular approach works.

Conventional psychiatric workers would like to use—and have consistently used—the double-blind study to determine the effectiveness of megavitamin therapy. The double-blind study has been, for the better part of the century, the experimental method of choice in virtually every field of medicine. There are a number of reasons for this. One is that medicine often has to deal with a disease in which the symptoms and changes in symptoms are very subtle. The corollary to this is that drugs developed to deal with these symptoms are just as subtle in their effects on the symptoms. Pharmaceutical houses spend millions of dollars developing drugs whose effect in some illnesses is so subtle it takes major statistical analyses performed with computers to determine whether or not the drug is indeed effective. "It is sometimes impossible to come up with convincing data," Dr. Kaufman says. "You can spend twenty years trying to figure out whether there is a difference between the drug and a sugar pill. The drug companies have the best statisticians money can buy and they spend all their time pumping data into computers to prove that a new compound has a remote chance of being significant. They'll fight tooth and nail with the FDA whether a drug has an effect or not.''

The underlying reason for all this is that the human mind has a tremendous effect on the way we react to medical attention. No one is exempt from this curious reaction to medication, not even the very scientists who should know better because they deal every day in very hard-nosed physiological research. "There is a man right here who has been shown that there is absolutely nothing wrong with his thyroid," Dr. Kaufman says, talking about a fellow researcher at NIH. "But once they took his thyroxine away from him and he was in bed dying. They gave the medicine back to him, and he's fine again. He's crazy, but he has to have his thyroxine."

"People just don't realize the potency of psychotherapy, that the mere fact of giving something has an enormous therapeutic value," Dr. Henry Borsook, a noted nutritionist at the University of California at Berkeley, says. "During the war, we did a study at Lockheed to see if giving workers vitamins in amounts greater than the recommended amount would make any difference to their health or performance. The experiment ran for a year and we examined them at the beginning, in the middle, and at the end. Half of the workers got placebos. We had gone through several hundred placebo pills, and a number of the workers who had been getting them asked me where they could buy these pills because they were getting so much good out of them and wanted to give them to their families. You have to see it to appreciate how potent the psychotherapeutic effect of getting a pill is."

It is, as Dr. Kaufman says, sometimes impossible to determine whether or not a new drug is any more effective than a sugar pill, a placebo. But, despite the difficulties, the attempt must be made, and the best way to do it, most researchers feel, is through the double-blind experiment. An experimental group of patients is divided into two groups. A batch of pills is prepared. Half the pills contain the placebo, the other half the new drug under scrutiny. Each batch has a code number—it wouldn't do, after all, to mark one bottle "Placebo" and the other "New Drug." Each patient is given a coded sample. The study is called double-blind, not because there are two sets of pills given, but because the experimenters who observe the patients, give them medical exams, and supervise laboratory tests don't know either which patients are getting the placebo and which the drug. At the end of the experimental period, the researchers tally up their observations on each individual patient, summarizing changes for the better, changes for the worse. The code is then broken and it is determined which patient was getting what. If it turns out that those receiving the drug had a significantly higher rate of measurable positive changes than those getting the placebo, the drug is on its way to acceptance.

Since the days of Freud, psychiatrists and psychologists have been struggling to gain acceptance as scientists, as thinkers whose propositions, theorems, and treatment approaches are true scientific precepts, not just philosophical spinnings. It is for this reason that, over the years, psychiatric researchers have struggled to find ways of making their beliefs and treatment methods "operational," to make them fit the same standards for scientific acceptability that are applied to other medical approaches. The struggle has been especially intense on the part of those psychiatrists who are seeking the biochemical roots and the biochemical solutions to mental illness. It is for these reasons that many psychiatric researchers insist on using the double-blind study to test concepts in the field of psychiatry. If megavitamin therapy is to be accepted as a tool in psychiatry, it must, critics say, pass the double-blind test.

But the orthomolecular psychiatrists do not buy the argument. "The double-blind study is a holy cow that everybody worships and which is totally inapplicable to psychiatric illness," Dr. Hawkins says. "It's a scientific method applicable to white rats in a laboratory environment in which all the variables are controlled and not to schizophrenics where you have an untold number of biochemical variables, age differences, dietary differences, family differences, differences over which you have no control."

Double-blind studies, say the orthomolecular psychiatrists, are essentially immoral. At the very least, they deprive the half of the experimental group that is receiving the placebo of a medicine that could help them. And, because many double-blind studies last a long time, they deny the drug to thousands of people who will fall ill or whose illness will worsen during the duration of a test that would only confirm that the drug is worthwhile. Dr. Osmond, for example, criticized a proposed four-year double-blind study at the New Jersey State Hospital because during the length of that study at least 200,000 young people would develop schizophrenia. "What is their fate, using every treatment known today, excluding niacin, likely to be?" Osmond asked. "Between 35 percent and 40 percent (70,000 to 80,000 patients) will recover from their initial illness which may last from some weeks to several years. After this they will not have a recurrence. About 30 percent (60,000 patients) will have one or more attacks of schizophrenia requiring further treatment in hospital during their lifetime. At the end of the four years we would expect that about 10 percent, that is, 15,000 to 20,000, of the original patients to be in some kind of a psychiatric hospital. There will have been about 105,000 admissions, resulting in some 26,900 years spent in hospital. Because the suicide rate for patients with schizophrenia . . . is about twenty times that of healthy people of the same age, between 750 and 1,000 of them will commit suicide during the four years." Megavitamins work, the orthomolecularists say. Why risk such a burdensome toll just to fulfill some musty scientific belief in double-blind studies?

To the orthomolecularists, the opposition to megavitamin treatment by establishment psychiatrists is strictly political: orthomolecular psychiatry threatens conventional psychiatrists. Therefore the immediate reaction is not to consider its virtues but to stamp it out before it destroys lifelong, comfortable treatment habits, before it undermines traditional, lucrative sources of income. "Psychiatry itself is controversial," Dr. Hawkins says. "And within psychiatry every mode of treatment is controversial. But the American Psychiatric Association has taken on megavitamin therapy as a project to put down at every opportunity. There have been papers written by prestigious psychiatrists that show that psychotherapy does nothing whatsoever for acute and chronic schizophrenics, but those papers were couched in language that would not offend their colleagues. So did every psychiatrist in the United States stop practicing psychotherapy with their patients? They did not. Did the APA put out a big polemic editorial blasting psychotherapy of schizophrenic patients? They did not.

"But the APA did write a blistering, extraordinarily biased editorial against the American Schizophrenic Association and this was long before there were any negative studies about orthomolecular psychiatry.

"Don't forget. The average orthomolecular psychiatrist can take on several hundred patients using this method as opposed to what he could carry if he gives each patient two or three weekly sessions of psychotherapy. If half a dozen or more orthomolecular psychiatrists suddenly start to practice in a community, the other psychiatrists are going to be affected."

The financial argument, of course, galls traditional psychiatrists. Says one, "I have referred half a dozen or so patients who requested it to orthomolecular psychiatrists. They tell me that the first visit cost them $25 to $35, and that included a visit with the nurse, taking the HOD test, and then seeing the doctor for the last ten minutes while he writes out the prescription for the vitamins. That means that the doctor can see four to six patients an hour. I have a hunch that these psychiatrists make $150 an hour. It's cheap for the patient all right, but more lucrative for the therapist. And sometimes I am not so sure it is cheaper for the patient. I have sent two ambulatory schizophrenics up to one of them who told me that they wanted the megavitamin therapy because they didn't have the money for my treatment. In both cases they came back and said that they were told they would have to go to the hospital and that would cost them $1,000 a week until they were under control." In any case, say the critics, the entire argument that traditionalists oppose megavitamin therapy because it would displace lucrative sources of income doesn't wash. Very few schizophrenics, the critics say, are still being treated with psychotherapy, and the number of psychiatrists practicing just psychotherapy on schizophrenics has greatly declined in the last few years.

The emotional appeal of megavitamin therapy is considerable. There is, after all, something very romantic about thinking that people crippled by serious mental illnesses that have defied traditional approaches can be cured through the faithful application of inexpensive (or, at least, theoretically inexpensive) vitamins and careful adherence to special diets. But once emotional appeal is put aside, there remain some serious doubts.

Perhaps one of the more troublesome aspects of megavitamin therapy is indeed the way a once relatively simple theory has, over the years, grown into a vastly complex edifice, a structure designed and built by a baroque architect gone mad. When Dr. Hoffer began his work with nicotinic acid, it was the vitamin and the vitamin alone that was given credit for the startling recovery made by people diagnosed as schizophrenic under Hoffer's care. Now, twenty years later, one can hardly discern the nicotinic acid for all the other vitamins, diets, and supplementary drugs that now accompany it. Orthomolecular psychiatrists argue that the adjuvant vitamins and diets are necessary and have increased their allegedly phenomenal treatment successes because, in the last few years, they have come to recognize that schizophrenia is a complicated disease. "Within the field of schizophrenia there are many subtypes [of the disease]," says Dr. Michael Lesser, a board-certified psychiatrist who now concentrates on nutritional approaches to the mental illness. "Seven different vitamin deficiencies will result in schizophrenia. As we learn more, the treatment has become more complex. To measure [the effectiveness] of this program, you need [wholly new] ways of studying it." And yet it is impossible to get away from the fact that Dr. Hoffer's original claim was that nicotinic acid, given in sufficient quantities, would help 75 percent of all schizophrenics. No orthomolecular psychiatrist I talked to, no matter how intricate his treatment methods, claimed he could top this figure.

Orthomolecular psychiatrists might argue—and they do—that each schizophrenic is an individual case, that a special vitamin regimen must be designed for every schizophrenic that walks through the office door. But again, Dr. Hoffer's original enthusiasm for nicotinic acid was based on his alleged success in treating people he broadly characterized as schizophrenic. Hoffer told of no specialized, involved biochemical tests, no extensive interviewing that sought to establish if Peter were different from P.F. or P.F. from Daniel. They were all schizophrenics, pure and simple, as far as he was concerned. And the regimen prescribed for them was nicotinic acid, pure and simple. No fancy footwork there. Furthermore, Dr. Hoffer has advocated that every person—whatever the state of their health—take one gram of nicotinic acid a day from infancy on, to safeguard against schizophrenia. He has made no similar recommendations for other vitamins.

It is, in other words, very, very hard to escape the conclusion that the addition of laver after layer of new supplemental ingredients to megavitamin therapy is not the work of an architect carefully working to build a flawless, well-integrated structure but that of a builder who is not quite sure what wind or load stresses his building will be able to weather, or what kind of a design the client really wants, and who therefore slaps on support after support, facade after facade, hoping that somehow the conglomeration will pass muster.

Those who have questioned megavitamin therapy have consistently wondered why there has been so much continuing dependence on nonorthomolecular methods like ECT. Many, if not most, traditional therapists long ago abandoned this therapy because they do not consider it very helpful in the long run and because it is essentially barbaric. Even Dr. Pauling, speaking before a symposium of orthomolecular experts, gently denounced electric-convulsive therapy as "closely analogous to a method of treatment of mental disease that I think was used traditionally by primitive man, that of hitting the patient over the head with a club."

Dr. Lesser, who practices in Berkeley, California, shrugs off ECT's role in orthomolecular therapy. "The use of ECT is a result of a generation gap," Lesser told me in the course of a telephone interview in May 1983. "Hoffer does it. Hawkins does it. But they are older men. I don't do it and most of the younger psychiatrists (who practice orthomolecular methods) don't use it."

Nevertheless, not only does Hoffer, the father of orthomolecular therapy, use ECT, but has encouraged its use, even roundly excoriating his opponents for not including it in their experiments to test megavitamin therapy. In fact, to a layman, Dr. Hoffer's enthusiasm for ECT can sometimes border on the frightening. In one paper, discussing the side effects of nicotinic acid, Dr. Hoffer went so far as to suggest that ECT could somehow short-circuit a patient's negative reactions to nicotinic acid. One patient, he said, could not take even one gram a day of nicotinic acid or nicotinamide because the vitamin made him vomit. Tranquilizers seemed to have the same effect on the patient. Yet, Dr. Hoffer said, the patient "took a series of electroconvulsant therapy and since has been able to take 6 gm of nicotinic acid per day without nausea and vomiting." The cruel implications of the statement are disturbing. Of course a patient who has had some kind of an aversion (remembering that mentally disturbed patients often get bizarre notions about what they eat or what they are given in the form of medication) to swallowing something strange will decide after a number of ECT treatments that it might not be a bad idea to take the damn stuff being offered him rather than go through another session with the electricity. I would imagine that a good many well-adjusted people would drink lye after receiving a series of ECT.

In fact, studying some of Dr. Hoffer's work with nicotinic acid and ECT, one has to wonder just why he credits nicotinic acid, not ECT, with some of the results he attributes to the nicotinic acid.[1] "One girl recently came up here from Texas to be treated," Dr. Hoffer said recently. "She had spent the past three years in a private psychiatric institution where she received group psychotherapy and perhaps a few drugs. Throughout that time she was constantly hallucinating on a rock singer who had died some time ago.

"The hospital staff at the end of three years had pretty well given up and did not know what more to do. Her father brought her up. She was started on the orthomolecular approach on Saturday. On Monday she had her first shock treatment. On Tuesday she was normal. For the first time in three years she stopped hallucinating. She received seven ECT treatments on the principle that too few are of no value and that the symptoms can return. She went home exactly four weeks after she was admitted, well for the first time in four years."

Finally, there seems to be no real proof that would tend to confirm the biochemical picture orthomolecular psychiatrists hold of schizophrenia. One of the major theories proposed by the megavitamin enthusiasts is that schizophrenia is induced by the presence of the aberrant adrenalinelike substance adrenochrome. Yet this substance has never been found in the human body. Furthermore, researchers say, in the normal human body one can measure a constant ratio among the various compounds that are members of the adrenaline family. If the process in which adrenaline is being

---

[1] The APA wonders too. "It is barely possible," the APA report notes, "that [ECT] may be [one of the] crucial variables [in the orthomolecular approach]. . . . If this should prove to be the case, the ECT may again deserve a place in the conventional treatment of schizophrenia."

formed (from noradrenaline, its predecessor substance) or if the process in which the adrenaline itself is being broken down were in some way going astray, a change in the normal values of the ratio among the various compounds involved would be easily distinguished. In fact, researchers say, they have found that the ratio among these compounds is no different in schizophrenics than in normal people.

Orthomolecular psychiatrists also like to argue that schizophrenia represents a nutritional disease, a spectacular sort of a deficiency, one that is genetically limited to one organ of the body, the brain. They point out that mental illness was rampant among victims of pellagra in the South during the early part of the century. They also like to point out that a researcher at Yale University has identified a host of inborn metabolic errors revolving about a genetic inability to utilize certain vitamins properly.

Critics rightly point out that while there are many diseases like pellagra that have a psychological component, the psychological aspect of the deficiency disease is rarely seen independent of other physical manifestations. Physiological problems might arise without being accompanied by psychological disturbances, but not the other way around, at least in no disease doctors know about. "The number of people suffering from pellagra who did not have physical symptoms like diarrhea and who were only crazy was very small," Dr. Lipton points out. "In every other case of vitamin deficiency or dependence, the patient will show manifestations other than just psychological ones. And, if ninety-nine vitamin diseases show a physical manifestation, I would expect the one hundredth to show them also. Schizophrenia would have to be the one exception."

Comparing schizophrenia to other vitamin-deficiency problems that are the result of inborn metabolic errors is also misleading. Those diseases have a host of characteristics that schizophrenia does not have: they are passed on from generation to generation in a clear, indisputable pattern; they appear almost as soon as the child is born; the child that has one of the diseases can be tested for an undisputed chemical aberration in the bloodstream; often they make themselves very apparent through a dramatic physiological event like anemia, mental retardation, or convulsions. Although some kind of a genetic component is suspected in schizophrenia. the disease has yet to yield clear-cut proof that it is strictly of hereditary origin. There are no universally accepted, indisputable blood or urine tests for schizophrenia. There are, again, no purely physiological manifestations, like convulsions, that can indisputably be linked to a metabolic problem concurrent with schizophrenia. But perhaps much more important, when a child with one of the recognized metabolic diseases is identified, a quick and massive application of the appropriate vitamin solves the problem virtually overnight. Absolutely nothing else—no other drugs, no other vitamins, no other additional and specialized diets—is required.

It is almost impossible not to conclude that those who practice orthomolecular psychiatry on their mentally ill and emotionally disturbed patients are dealing not with hard-and-fast schizophrenics but either with borderline schizophrenics, or neurotics, or both. The conclusion can be reached not just from the more carefully controlled studies that have failed to support the claims of the orthomolecularists, but it can also be reached just by talking to some of the patients who say they have been helped by megavitamins.

I asked Dr. Harvey Ross, who is recognized as one of the leading practitioners of orthomolecular therapy, to introduce me to some of his patients, the ones he has treated successfully with megavitamins. Every one of the patients (or every one of the parents of one of his patients) was enthusiastic about Dr. Ross, his therapeutic approach, and the results achieved. But, as more and more of them called me, a disturbing pattern became apparent: few had really ever been given a clear-cut and unquestioned diagnosis of schizophrenia.

Robert Applegate, a construction worker, told me that Dr. Ross's megavitamin approach now allowed him to live a full life for the first time in years. He had had repeated bouts of mental illness, including four different hospitalizations, ranging in length from several days to several months, before he found Dr. Ross. During one of those hospitalizations, Applegate told me, he was diagnosed as schizophrenic. On another occasion, he was told that he was manic-depressive. Dr. Ross, Applegate says, tested him for hypoglycemia but never told him that he is schizophrenic. "Dr. Ross put me on a special diet and prescribed 4,500 milligrams of niacin, 1,600 international units of vitamin E, 1,500 milligrams of

C, pantothenic acid, B complex, and some other nutrients and minerals," Applegate says. "I sleep better, I don't get palpitations whenever someone talks to me, and I can communicate and talk with people. I can even go on a date now."

Mrs. Annette DiGiorgio says that she went to Dr. Ross almost as a last resort. For most of her adult life (she is now forty and her problems began when she was nineteen), Mrs. DiGiorgio says, she had been having all sorts of medical problems. Yet, whenever she went to see a doctor, thorough examinations failed to reveal any underlying physiological causes. She also suffered severe anxiety attacks. "I couldn't even take the garbage out," she says. "I had to give up driving. If I had to go to the supermarket, I'd start hyperventilating and get dizzy. I never gave the kids a bath unless my husband was home because I was afraid I'd lose control and kill them. There weren't ten minutes in those years that I felt normal.

"I went to a local mental health center to get help and got into group therapy for six months, but that was of no help. I went with my husband to get counseling, and that didn't help. I saw a psychiatrist for six years but got no better.

"Then I saw an article about low blood sugar and that it could cause some of the problems I had been having. And I also saw an article by Dr. Pauling, so I wrote him and asked him to recommend an orthomolecular psychiatrist. He wrote back and recommended Dr. Ross."

Dr. Ross, Mrs. DiGiorgio says, gave her a number of tests, including one for hypoglycemia. "He put me on the low-blood-sugar diet and started me on the vitamins. I felt terrible at first, the diet made me feel bad. I had ups and downs, but after a while the downs started not to be so down and the good times got better. Two weeks ago I drove again for the first time in fifteen years."

One of Dr. Ross's patients is another young man whom another orthomolecular psychiatrist had labeled a schizophrenic after a short interview. The boy—let's call him David—had been a hyperactive child, who had had trouble learning to read and who, since the age of six, had been treated with Stelazine and Ritalin. "We took him to the first psychiatrist when he started hearing voices," David's mother says, recounting his most recent problems. "The doctor gave him twenty-six shock treatments, gave him vitamins and tranquilizers. After all that, David was still hearing voices and the psychiatrist said he couldn't understand why he hadn't improved. He just dropped him like a hot potato.

"We put him in a second hospital where they kept him heavily medicated all the time. It got to the point where he was so overloaded with tranquilizers that he couldn't even sit up. Now as far as I know, David wasn't given any tests, but the second doctor told us that he saw no hope at all for David and that he would have to stay in the hospital indefinitely.

"Then we heard about Dr. Ross. Dr. Ross took him off all the medication immediately, but did put him on a very mild dose of a tranquilizer and another drug to offset a bit the effects of the tranquilizers. He put him on 4,500 milligrams of niacin, 3,000 milligrams of C, 1,200 international units of E, 600 milligrams of B_6, 300 milligrams of pantothenic acid, 500 milligrams of B complex, 1,800 milligrams of l-glutamine, 25 milligrams of potassium, and the hypoglycemic diet.

"The change was slow at first, but now we see that David has made a remarkable recovery. Last summer he couldn't rake a leaf off the lawn, last week he weeded my garden. He is playing basketball and football again, and he is slowly getting his coordination back. He is still not entirely well, but he is so much better that it's like a miracle."

There can be very little doubt that Dr. Ross and other orthomolecular psychiatrists are achieving results with people who have significant emotional problems. But if the vitamins are not responsible for the recoveries, what is?

The most likely explanation is that orthomolecular psychiatrists are practicing an artful and successful form of psychotherapy on their patients. "These are people who are either borderline schizophrenics or who are generally not as crazy," says Dr. Loren Mosher, chief of the Center for the Study of Schizophrenia at the National Institute of Mental Health. "It is easier to make them better." In other words, orthomolecular psychiatrists by and large see people who, although mentally ill, are amenable to suggestion, who can be made to believe that this highly intricate therapy will work. Just as there are people who get relief from aspirin but not Anacin (and vice versa), there are people who benefit from orthomolecular psychiatry when all other approaches have failed.

Orthomolecular psychiatrists, of course, don't agree. "You

can't rule out the milieu, the experience of the individuals,'' Dr.
Weathers says. ''But the proof of the pudding is in the clinical
response of the patients. You take a blatantly psychotic individual
who has been maintained on phenothiazines and is still hallucinating and having delusions, you take care of the hypoglycemic state
and his vitamin deficiencies, and in a matter of weeks this individual is freed of hallucinations, is returned to work, is at home and is
functional. It is a beautiful thing to see how they improve when
they follow instructions.''

No one can fairly say, argues Dr. Ross, that it is the psychiatrist's magnetic personality that is mesmerizing the patient into getting better. ''We all have had patients, not many, whom we have
had to treat without seeing because of some extraordinary circumstance. I treated one young man this way, the only one I have done
this way because it is not a good idea, who was in his early thirties.
He was a playwright in New York and he had developed a paranoid
schizophrenia that kept him in the house, unable to work. He had
three voices going at him all the time. He had tremendous pains all
the time. He said the voices were preventing him from moving his
bowels.

''His girl friend came to me for advice because she said she had
been reading about megavitamins. She went around getting all the
vitamins and gave them to him for three months. He didn't know
he was getting anything, but after a few months he started to improve and was willing to get out of the apartment to come see me.
Several months later he was out again, writing again. He started to
get well before he saw me.''

Ross stops his monologue for a moment. We are talking in his
office in a spacious suite just off Sunset Boulevard on the edge of
Los Angeles, just across the street from Beverly Hills. He is a
young man, good-looking, and could just as well be sitting down-
stairs at Schwab's, drinking the proverbial milk shake, waiting for
the proverbial Hollywood talent scout. We've been talking for a
while and he seems somewhat saddened by the challenges to the
type of medicine he practices. He glances at his watch—there is a
young man outside taking a test under the supervision of the recep-
tionist—and goes on talking.

''Unfortunately,'' he says, tracing the tips of his fingers over
the long surface of the massive desk, ''it's gotten to the point

where no one believes anyone anymore.

"The problem is that we accepted the criticisms as a challenge, as an attack. So we attacked back. That gets you in a position where you start to make claims you shouldn't be making, or saying that this is better than it really is. We should have been saying, look, buddy, we are both working toward the same thing, how can we work together, rather than fight one another."

The "other" psychiatrists don't sympathize at all. What the orthomolecular therapists have done, the critics say, is not just gotten themselves into a position where they are making claims they shouldn't be making, but gotten themselves into a position where they just cannot understand what kind of medicine they are really practicing. Some critics maintain that these therapists just don't understand that they are helping their patients not because they are practicing a form of psychotherapy or hypnosis but because they are practicing a very subtle form of corrective medicine. In many instances, some skeptics say, the orthomolecular psychiatrists are not correcting some theoretical abnormality in the molecular composition of the brain but are correcting the harm done by other psychiatrists who are much too free with conventional drugs.

"You see, what happens is that you have some guy who is not adjusting well, so some psychiatrist goes and diagnoses him as schizophrenic and fills him full of drugs," Dr. Edward T. Yorke, staff psychiatrist at Camarillo State Hospital near Los Angeles, says. "With those drugs, the doctor has reduced the patient's spontaneity of thinking. The patient loses his ability to carry out abstract functions. He is too lethargic to make any effort. He does not engage in goal-directed behavior. He can't remember things. They keep guys stupid like this for six or eight years and cause the very problem they are trying to treat. In other words, you have diagnosed him badly, you put him on drugs, and you make him act just like a schizophrenic."

Yorke pauses to let the point sink in. Outside his office—a small room whose walls have long ago lost their institutional coloring to the onslaughts of dirt and perhaps an occasional ray of sun—one can hear the murmurings of the deeply disturbed men he is treating. Yorke himself looks tired, a bit beaten down by the long years he has put in, trying to care for psychotics, the mentally retarded, the abandoned senile in this state-supported institution. He wears old clothes, a suit that has seen better days, a shirt open at the collar.

"So someone finally comes along and takes this guy to an orthomolecular psychiatrist," he is saying as I study him. "The first thing he does is take the guy off all that junk, and the patient immediately gets better. That is what may be helping, not the megavitamins."

Yorke gets up to walk me out of the ward. "When I first came to Camarillo," Yorke is saying, fishing for the keys that will unlock the doors, "everyone thought I was a genius. I was going into wards, making changes in the medication, and suddenly all these patients were getting better, starting to snap out of their lethargy, actually seeing what they were staring at on the tube. They all thought I was prescribing some new combinations of drugs. I wasn't. I was just cutting in half all the stuff that had been prescribed by the doctors before I came along."

I remember Dr. Yorke's explanations as Dr. Ross's patients tell me of their experiences with megavitamins. "I snapped back in the early part of 1972," Jerry, an electrician, tells me. "I had been working long hours, I was going to school, and I was having trouble with my girlfriend, getting engaged, breaking off the engagement. I started to see a psychiatrist and he had me strung out bad on Valium, Librium, Thorazine, Stelazine. The combination was really deadly and it got to the point where I was one hell of a mess. I mean, I was a vegetable. I stayed in my room for a year.

"Then I read in the *Los Angeles Times* about megavitamin therapy and the article listed some of the symptoms of schizophrenia that I thought paralleled what I was going through. I went to see Dr. Ross and he gave me a lot of tests and told me that I was suffering a latent schizophrenia. He started me on megavitamins and put me on a low-dosage tranquilizer. I snapped right out of it and the whole thing disappeared like a bad dream. Every day is fine now."

The orthomolecularists, convinced that they are right, naturally shrug off all the explanations. "They say, well, people who are helped maybe are not schizophrenic," Dr. Ross says. "But the people who were helped, whatever you call them, came to a psychiatrist because they were ill, they were suffering. Even in implying that these people are not schizophrenic, they say that we helped them.''

The argument, however, cannot be dismissed as lightly as that. To imply that people, whatever they are labeled, are helped anyway by megavitamins, so why quibble, is to imply that the treatment is effective across the board, that orthomolecular psychiatry has no negative fallout whatsoever. That, however, is just not true. It is true that many psychiatrists using the orthomolecular approach show genuine concern for their patients. The North Nassau Mental Health Center has an assortment of ancillary services—hospitalization, family services, halfway house, access to support activities like Schizophrenics Anonymous for the patient—which even the APA admits represent a giant step forward in the provision of mental health care. Many patients who come to the center stand an excellent chance of receiving the kind of attention and the kind of intensive personal care that could in itself help them cope with mental illness. Dr. Ross too, as far as I could see, and Dr. Weathers provide some personal support for their patients. But in surveying the orthomolecular field and in talking to many of those who practice in it, I got the uncomfortable feeling that an overwhelming majority of the psychiatrists have a good many patients who come to them, whom they see briefly while they are writing out the prescription for the megavitamins and whom they may see only sporadically for an occasional chat or checkup. Many of these psychiatrists see patients who come to them from distant places, who get their prescriptions for the vitamins and then go back where they came from, never to be seen again.

It seems to me that it is grossly irresponsible to give a patient a vitamin prescription, a prescription for a low-dose tranquilizer, and a mimeographed sheet outlining a special diet, and to assume that that is all he needs. If a fair portion of seriously disturbed individuals do find their way to orthomolecular psychiatrists, how can these practitioners blithely assume that they need nothing more than a bottle of pills? ''Imagine,'' suggests Dr. Loren Mosher, ''a man of forty whose mother has been surreptitiously spiking his orange juice with LSD for the past twenty-five years. Suddenly the mother dies, and the morning of her funeral her bereaved son's biochemical peculiarity is suddenly corrected. Could we really expect this man to pick up a hat and briefcase and head downtown for his first day on the job? One suspects that psychological therapy and retraining would be vital in helping this poor fellow match his behavior pattern to his newfound biochemical normality.''

It is imaginable, is it not, that the emotionally unstable person who has recovered under the belief that vitamins are realigning the molecules in his brain would, like Mosher's fictional LSD victim, need some help in readjusting to the "real" world? He would. But it seems that even the best-intentioned of orthomolecular psychiatrists do not understand this. Ruby, the Toronto woman who came to Los Angeles, told me plaintively that megavitamins had helped her regain some stability. But she also told me that she felt she still had a long way to go—that her mind "still goes blank" during interviews, that she has yet to make a full adjustment to the world around her. How often does she see Dr. Ross, I asked her? "Oh, only every two months or so," she said. "I'd like to see him more but I really can't afford to see him more than that now."

The feeling is virtually unavoidable that orthomolecular therapy is an unfortunate mutant that has been conceived, raised, and unleashed on the world by people whose capacity for wishful thinking has exceeded their capacity for sagacious scientific work. A theory—that nicotinic acid could be a prime therapeutic agent against schizophrenia—was formulated in a rush of excitement. The very gleam of the idea mesmerized its originators, who worked hard to make their theory a self-fulfilling prophecy. Others, anxious to join in this exciting development that could spare the minds of millions, joined in their pet theories and beliefs. At the end of it all, there has emerged a curious amalgam of scientific possibility and folk medicine.

The truly unfortunate part is that if orthomolecular psychiatrists and theoreticians had been a little less anxious to rush out and announce their ideas to the world, they might have carried out the kind of scientific experiments that might conceivably have proven the worthiness of their theories (if indeed they did have any potential for scientific validity). The possibility still exists, after all—and no one, not even Dr. Ban nor Dr. Lipton, would deny it—that vitamins may play some role in mental illness. But if that possibility exists, it would have to be ferreted out by proper work.

If, as some argue convincingly, schizophrenia is not a single disease but is a symptom common to many different mental disturbances, careful studied work with nicotinic acid might have uncovered just one of the many processes that might be behind the ill-ness. The process might be at work in 1, 2, 5 percent of all schizophrenics. To find that nicotinic acid really helps 5 percent of the schizophrenic population might not have been very much. But it would have represented a meaningful start of a meaningful offen-sive against the disease. The orthomolecularists, however, would not have been content to have attained so modest an achievement. They had to try to prove to the world that megavitamins are effec-tive in the great majority of all schizophrenic cases. In the process they proved nothing at all, wasting a lot of time, money, and scien-tific energy.

CHAPTER VII

Everyman's Vitamin

"But what about my vitamin C?" asks the still-sleepy, befuddled father in the television commercial as a mysterious new breakfast drink makes its debut on his kitchen nook table. Not to worry, his wife assures him in the midst of the morning-meal bedlam that surrounds him, there is as much C in this new potion as there is in "that other breakfast drink." A little more awake now, but looking not very much smarter, the good man takes his glass and drinks. Smiling with great satisfaction because he has been assured that for another twenty-four hours he is protected against the ravages of scurvy, he fades into the next fifteen minutes of *Sunday Night at the Movies*.

There are a few million people here and there who worry that without vitamin E they are more likely to drop dead from a heart attack. A few million are convinced that their diets, poor in nicotinic acid, are paving the way for them to the local insane asylum. But tens of millions who would scoff and snicker at the nuts who swallow vitamin pills and capsules by the handful would themselves not dare venture into the day without their morning ration of ascorbic acid, vitamin C. Ascorbic acid, after all, is the elder statesvitamin of nutrition. It is the one vitamin with a clearly proven track record more than four hundred years old, the one vitamin clearly linked, in the public's eye, with a devastating disease bearing a terrifying name, scurvy.

"The signes to know this disease in the beginning are divers, by the swelling of the gummes, by denting of the flesh of the leggs with a man's finger, the pit remaining without filling up in a good space," Sir Richard Hawkins wrote in his *Observations* of his voyage to the South Sea in 1593. "Others show it with their lasinesse, others complaine of the ricke of the backe, etc, all which are for the most part certaine tokens of infection. . . ."

Scurvy was, and still is, a devastating disease. The illness starts with fatigue and aching of the arms and legs. Sufferers feel a vague malaise, just not feeling up to par. In time, the scurvy patient develops a few spots on the legs, spots that are really signs of small subskin hemorrhages called petechiae. In time, as the disease becomes more virulent, its signs become more severe as well. Gums may start bleeding and hemorrhages begin striking the eyes. Glands that secrete fluids—notably the tear glands and salivary glands—dry up. As the disease progresses, the hemorrhages spread. Uncontrolled bleeding under the covering over the nerves results in a buildup of pressures that cause the nerves to malfunction. There is a marked drop in urine output, and water starts accumulating in the legs. Hemorrhages spread to the muscles and intestines. Depression and arthritis set in.

"The cause of this sickness," Sir Richard observed in his 1593 book, "some attribute to sloath, some to conceite, and divers men speak diversly. . . . That which I have seen most fruitful for this sickness, is sower Oranges and Lemmons. . . ." Eight years later, in 1601, Sir James Lancaster ordered that all ships sailing under the charter of the East India Company carry fruit juices, which were to be part of the sailors' daily diets. Despite Sir Richard Hawkins's insight into a simple cure for scurvy, the disease went largely unchecked. In 1593, the very year Sir Richard wrote that "sower Oranges and Lemmons" were effective antidotes to scurvy, ten thousand British soldiers died of the disease. In 1740, 139 years after Sir James's edict to the private trading company's captains, Admiral George Anson, also an Englishman, set out to show the British flag with a six-ship squadron and 961 sailors. Within a year almost half of his men had died of scurvy.

James Lind, a Scottish physician serving in the British navy, is generally credited with initiating the movement to gain citrus fruits recognition as effective anti-scurvy agents. Goaded by an interest in

the disease and appalled by the toll taken by it, Lind first researched records of sea voyages. He found that the disease seemed
to cause no problems on ships plying the southern seas, ships carrying cargoes of fresh fruits, which the sailors ate liberally during
their long voyages.

Intrigued by the connection, Lind took twelve scurvy patients to
sea aboard the *Salisbury* and fed them different concoctions and
medications, including fresh fruit juices. If he were right, he theo-
rized, those scurvy patients given the fresh fruits would recover.
The others would not.

"Two of these," Lind wrote in his *A Treatise on the Scurvy,*
published in 1753, "were ordered each a quart of cyder a-day. Two
others took twenty-five gutts [drops] of elixir vitriol three times a
day, upon an empty stomach. . . . Two of the worst patients, with
the tendons in the ham rigid, were put under a course of sea-water.
Of this they drank half a pint a day, and sometimes more or less, as
it operated by way of gentle psychic. Two others had each two
oranges and one lemon given them every day. . . . They ate with
great greediness, at different times, upon an empty stomach. They
continued but six days under this course, having consumed the
quantity that could be spared. The two remaining patients took the
bigness of a nutmeg three times a-day, of an electuary recommended by an hospital-surgeon, made of garlic, mustard seed, . . .
balsam of Peru, and gum-myrrh; using for common drink barley
water." The consequences of the experiment were immediately apparent: The two scurvy patients given the plain citrus fruits recovered within six days and were well enough to help tend the other
patients. The others, as Lind had predicted, did not recover on their
assorted prescriptions.

Despite Lind's experiment, there was no immediate and univer-
sal move to include fresh fruits in the food stocks of ships going to
sea. The British navy, for example, did not enforce the use of foods
with antiscorbutic properties in shipboard menus until 1804. After
Lind had conducted his experiments and after it had been recommended that lime juice, easily stored and carried, might be issued
to British sailors on the high seas, many of the men who were taking lime juice, skeptics discovered, were still coming down with
scurvy. The incidence of scurvy among these men, Lind's critics
said, proved that foods had nothing to do with the disease. The

British navy relented only after it was discovered that those sailors who were still coming down with scurvy were doing so because they were boiling their lime juice (boiling, we now know, destroys the vitamin C in the juice) before taking it and only after Lind repeated his experiment, proving once more that fresh, uncooked fruits were indeed antiscorbutic. When Lind's recommendations were finally adopted, the benefits were immediate. While there had been almost fifteen hundred cases of scurvy under treatment in one British navy hospital in 1780, there was only one case reported under treatment in the same hospital in 1806.

As late as the very early 1900s, in fact, a number of scientists and nutrition researchers were still not convinced and were still arguing that fruits and vegetables had nothing to do with the presence or absence of scurvy. The disease, they maintained, was caused by constipation and a resultant increase of poisonous substances in the gastrointestinal tract, substances that found their way into the rest of the body, where they carried out their destructive functions. Autopsies on guinea pigs that had died of scurvy, it was argued, revealed that part of the intenstinal tract of these animals was full of petrifying feces. This was taken as obvious proof that poisoning of sorts caused scurvy because the animals had lost the mechanical ability to defecate properly. To put the argument finally to rest, other nutritionists sacrificed guinea pigs that had no scurvy and demonstrated that these animals also had high fecal contents in part of the intestinal tract. Furthermore, by sacrificing a large number of scorbutic animals, provitamin forces established that only a small percentage of the guinea pigs had actually been constipated at the moment of death. Early in this century, Norwegian experimenters carried out another conclusive experiment. Using guinea pigs that had been in apparently good health while on a normal diet, the experimenters then began feeding the animals only grain products. In time, the guinea pigs developed scurvy. The researchers then fed the guinea pigs fresh fruits and vegetables and watched with satisfaction as the disease quickly cleared up.

Once it had been established that fresh fruits and vegetables do indeed contain an agent that is effective against scurvy, researchers all over the world raced to identify the compound within the foods that was specifically responsible for the antiscorbutic effect. The most imaginative work—and the work that was ultimately to end in the identification of vitamin C—was done by a Hungarian biochemist, Albert Szent-Györgyi, who at the beginning of the search was only tangentially interested in vitamins. Actually he initially assigned research on the vitamin to a junior colleague in his lab. "Vitamins," Szent-Györgyi recalls, "were to my mind, theoretically uninteresting. Vitamins means that one has to eat it. What one has to eat is the first concern of the chef, not the scientist." The casual attitude did not prevent Szent-Györgyi from identifying a mysterious substance in the adrenal cortex of animals. The substance would ultimately prove to be vitamin C. But when Szent-Györgyi discovered it, he was not quite sure what it was, so he dubbed it "ignose," meaning more or less that he was ignorant of the true nature of this compound, which had some sugarlike characteristics. When Arthur Harden, the editor of the *Biochemical Journal*—the journal to which Szent-Györgyi had sent his article announcing his discovery—saw the name the Hungarian had given the substance, he sent back the article, giving Szent-Györgyi a stiff reprimand on his choice of nomenclature. Szent-Györgyi, not to be deterred, sent the paper back, changing "ignose" to "Godnose." Harden, willing to put up with an eccentric but brilliant Hungarian scientist, sent the paper back for one more attempt at a proper name. Szent-Györgyi came up with "hexuronic acid" and the paper was published.

Shortly after the publication of his paper announcing the discovery of "hexuronic acid," Szent-Györgyi isolated the substance in fruits and vegetables, including oranges, cabbages, and his own beloved Hungarian red peppers. Believing now that hexuronic acid might be the antiscorbutic agent, he fed the hexuronic acid to scorbutic guinea pigs and watched them recover. The province of the chef had suddenly become the province of the biochemist. Within five years, the precise chemical nature and qualities of the substance were worked out; it was renamed ascorbic acid and the world had one more vitamin to think about.

Continuing research into vitamin C yielded a trove of information. Scientists learned that ascorbic acid helps the body utilize iron. At the same time, ascorbic acid performs a vital role in the body by preventing the premature or excessive burning up of vitamins A and E and various vitamins in the B complex: thiamine, riboflavin, folic acid, and pantothenic acid. They learned that ascorbic acid is to be found in large concentrations in those tissues and glands that are active in the body's metabolism. Thus, while muscle tissue is relatively low in vitamin C, the pituitary gland, the adrenal cortex, the thymus, the liver, the brain, the testes, and the ovaries are suffused with ascorbic acid. Researchers found that vitamin C seems to be intimately involved in the production or release of a number of important hormones and compounds, including cortisone and norepinephrine. Vitamin C is also involved in the conversion of a substance known as tryptophan into another chemical compound called 5HT (5-hydroxy tryptamine). The compound 5HT, in turn, is ultimately turned into serotonin. And both serotonin and 5HT are powerful compounds that influence the activities of the various organs in the body.

There are, of course, many things researchers still do not know about vitamin C. Vitamin C enhances many of the body's metabolic reactions. Thus it would seem logical that an absence of vitamin C would then slow down, or maybe even stop, these metabolic reactions. But a lack of vitamin C does no such thing; the metabolic reactions go right on. What is C's precise role in metabolism? Vitamin C is important in the production of many key hormones, but when vitamin C is withdrawn from the diet and scurvy results, none of the symptoms of the disease can be traced to an absence or shortage of the hormones linked to vitamin C. For example, people with scurvy are often depressed and lethargic—but researchers have found no evidence of reduced levels of norepinephrine and serotonin (which are thought to influence mental and emotional upheavals) in scorbutic patients. Why, then, is C important to hormones?

Despite these and other unanswered questions, a number of doctors and nutritionists have looked to the vitamin in the hope that it might (either in massive doses or in doses no larger than those available in a good, well-rounded diet) be the answer for a number of human complaints. These hopes seem to be founded largely on the dramatic successes doctors had in treating scurvy with vitamin C. Since scurvy includes a vast number of physiological (and psychological) problems and since C is capable of curing scurvy, it has been reasoned, it is also possible that the vitamin is an effective cure for similar problems when the scurvy itself is not present.

Thus, over the years, vitamin C has been proposed as an effective cure-all for problems ranging from lethargy to systemic infections.

In a few instances, ascorbic acid has been found to be important in nonscurvy problems, including the proper healing of wounds. In the days when sailors were falling prey to scurvy during their long voyages to the Far East or the New World, scurvy was also causing a problem among fighting men. As early as the first Crusades, doctors noticed that soldiers who showed even slight signs of scurvy were slower to recover from wounds than their companions who were not scorbutic. In fact, accounts of European battles and wars, written by doctors or military historians, contain many passages detailing slower wound healing among soldiers who had symptoms of scurvy than among other healthier soldiers. "But a most extraordinary circumstance," wrote the Reverend Richard Walter, discussing the problem of wound healing among scorbutic British navy personnel, in the eighteenth century, "and what would be scarcely credible upon any single evidence, is that the scars of wounds which had for many years healed were forced open again by this violent distemper: Of this, there was a remarkable instance, in one of the invalids upon the 'Centurion,' who had been wounded above 50 years before at the battle of the Boyne: for though he was cured soon after, and had continued well for a great number of years past, yet on his being attacked by the scurvy, his wounds, in the progress of his disease, broke out afresh, and appeared as if they had never healed: Nay what is still more astonishing, the callus of a broken bone, which had been completely formed for a long time, was found to be thereby dissolved, and the fracture seemed as if it had never been consolidated."

The special problems engendered by wounds in people with low vitamin C intake were studied well into the twentieth century. According to Geoffrey H. Bourne, director of the Yerkes Primate Center in Atlanta, Georgia, and a leading expert on the vitamin, early experiments with guinea pigs proved conclusively that vitamin C is important not only in the formation of tissues that cover wounds but also in the formation of tissues that form to repair bone damage. Proper healing of small wounds or bone problems in laboratory animals, Dr. Bourne says, is accomplished with as little as 2 milligrams of C a day—the equivalent of 40 to 50 milligrams for an adult human being. During the Second World War, doctors in England used vitamin C aggressively. In the early part of the war, surgeons noticed that soldiers (and civilians as well) were recovering much too slowly from wounds. In time doctors realized that because of wartime shortages, rationing, and other restrictions, people were getting far too little vitamin C. As a result, the physicians ordered hospital diets improved to include more vitamin C and, in some cases, when wounds were extensive or very serious, ordered supplemental vitamin C to be administered to the wounded patient.

Vitamin C's role in proper wound healing is fairly well accepted. That it is important for other things remains controversial. Some doctors, noting ascorbic acid's importance in the formation of skin and bone tissues, have speculated that massive doses of vitamin C might help people who have back problems caused by weakened intervertebral discs. When these discs—which separate the bones that make up the spinal column—slip out of place or rupture, the thinking goes, vitamin C can help by strengthening the tissues that keep the discs in place or by actually helping in the repair of the discs themselves. Dr. James Greenwood, Jr., a clinical professor of neurosurgery at Baylor College of Medicine, has urged people with a history of back problems to take at least 500 milligrams of ascorbic acid a day routinely and up to 1,000 milligrams if they feel pains and aches coming on or if they are about to start some activity that will put undue strain on their backs. He is convinced, Dr. Greenwood has said, that people who take high doses of C have less muscular soreness after exercise than people who do not take C. "It can be stated with reasonable assurance," Dr. Greenwood has reported, "that a significant percentage of patients with early disc lesions were able to avoid surgery by the use of large doses of vitamin C. Many of these patients after a few months or years stopped their vitamin C and symptoms recurred. When they were placed back on the vitamin the symptoms disappeared. Some, of course, eventually came to surgery."

While the idea sounds good, it must be remembered that so-called back problems and disc problems are whimsical conditions that in many instances confound sufferer and physician alike. Some patients are plagued by back-related pain all their lives. Others have a single bout of back problems and never go through another attack for the rest of their lives. Still others—most back-problem patients, in fact—have recurring problems. Some of these sufferers know that lifting a heavy package will trigger back spasms. Others know that twisting suddenly will land them in bed with heat packs or with a traction pulley tugging at their hips. Others never know what it is that aggravates their condition—all they know is that from time to time the old corset (another anti-bad-back weapon) has to come out of the drawer. Any good physician will say that it is impossible to forecast what course any patient's bout with back problems will take, to say with any certainty what mode of treatment will allevi- ate the patient's sufferings. Some patients recover even though nothing is done. Some respond to traction, others don't. Some respond to simple bedrest, while others find it completely useless. Because the problem is so whimsical, few doctors will take a chance and say "this is the treatment that will work." To put it another way: one could just as well say that patients treated inter- mittently with traction are more likely to avoid surgery as one could say that patients taking vitamin C regularly can keep the surgical knife at bay. Given a large enough number of patients put into trac- tion for four hours a day every week, it would be just as easy in all probability to demonstrate that many of them too were able to avoid early surgery.

Vitamin C's role in relieving listlessness and fatigue is also questionable. Because one of the symptoms that accompanies scurvy is lethargy, some vitamin C advocates have urged that the vitamin be used in massive doses to give people more mental and physical energy. But again, observations on the matter are in- conclusive, if not entirely negative. One research team gave eighty- seven soldiers in basic training 1 gram of ascorbic acid every day for two months. Those soldiers were able to adapt no better to the rigors of boot camp than soldiers who went through basic training eating nothing more than the usual army fare. Researchers at Stan- ford University ran a double-blind study in which freshmen and sophomore medical students—people traditionally under a great deal of stress and anxiety and therefore in need of great stores of energy—were given 1,500 milligrams of vitamin C daily to test the theory that C in massive doses would help alleviate the strains of medical school work and endow the students with an extra measure of power to deal with the daily rigors of classes and study. The students were divided into two groups. One group received the high doses of vitamin C for one month, while a second group received a placebo. The following month, the students who had been receiving the ascorbic acid were given the placebo and the students who had been receiving the inert pill were given ascorbic acid (none of the students theoretically knew who was getting what). Each student was asked to fill out questionnaires about the state of his health during the two months of the study. Analysis of the questionnaires and other data, the researchers said, "clearly proved that ascorbic acid, given at a dose more than ten times greater than the minimum daily requirement, could not be distinguished from the placebo in its influence upon the mental or physical well-being of our subjects."

A number of doctors and researchers have tried to establish a link between ascorbic acid and the levels of cholesterol and other atherosclerosis-inducing fats in the bloodstream. An appropriate dose of ascorbic acid, some believe, will lower the amount of fat in the arteries and might even be responsible for dissolving atherosclerotic plaques already formed on key arteries around the body.

According to Dr. Emil Ginter, head of the Department of Biochemistry at the Institute of Human Nutrition in Bratislava, Czechoslovakia, ascorbic acid may well have a positive influence on blood cholesterol levels. According to Dr. Ginter, guinea pigs fed a high-fat, low-vitamin-C diet accumulate more cholesterol in various body tissues (including the liver) and the wall of the aorta than guinea pigs fed diets with a normal amount of C. At least in the case of the guinea pigs, Dr. Ginter believes, the ascorbic acid plays a key—but still undefined—role in breaking down cholesterol into bile acids. When the body does not get enough ascorbic acid, Dr. Ginter has proposed, the cholesterol is not broken down properly and instead accumulates in the body to the detriment of the animal.

Dr. Ginter and his associates have also proposed that moderate increases in ascorbic acid (up to 300 milligrams a day) can have a positive effect on the cholesterol levels in human beings. Ginter tested his theory on residents of four villages in Slovakia. The villagers were divided into two groups. One group received no vitamin C supplements. The other group received ascorbic acid (300 milligrams daily) for roughly seven weeks. According to Dr. Ginter, the cholesterol levels in both groups were practically the same at the beginning of the experiment. "The administration of vitamin C resulted in the experimental group in a slight, but statistically significant decrease of cholesterolemia," Ginter reported. The vitamin's effects, Dr. Ginter said, were most noticeable in those people whose blood cholesterol levels were above 240 milligrams of cholesterol per milliliter of blood. In one subject, whose cholesterol level approached the 300-milligram level (a level at which the risk of a heart attack is very high) before the experiment began, the drop in cholesterol was 92 milligrams after the increased vitamin C intake.

Dr. Constance Spittle in England has been one of the most active supporters of the belief that ascorbic acid can keep down cholesterol and that it might, as a result, protect people against cardiovascular problems brought on by fatty deposits inside artery walls. After she noticed that she could vary her own cholesterol levels by almost 100 milligrams by varying her ascorbic acid intake, Dr. Spittle says, she began an experiment to see if the vitamin had the same effect on anyone else. First she studied fifty-eight persons—hospital personnel and their relatives—who were considered to be in good health. After their serum cholesterol levels had been followed for six weeks, the fifty-eight volunteers were given 1 gram of vitamin C a day for another six weeks, while their blood cholesterol levels were again monitored. During this second six-week period, among those volunteers under the age of twenty-five cholesterol levels tended to fall somewhat as a result of the vitamin C intake. Volunteers between the ages of twenty-five and forty-five, Dr. Spittle says, showed little change. The volunteers over the age of forty-five showed no consistent patterns, though some did show a *rise* in the serum cholesterol level after they had been on the ascorbic-acid regimen. Once the results from this group of fifty-eight were in, the experiment was repeated in twenty-five patients who had atherosclerosis and who had had heart attacks. In this group, Dr. Spittle reports, the effects of the vitamin C were striking: there was a significant increase in the *rise* of serum cholesterol in the blood.

There are adequate explanations for the *fall* in cholesterol levels in the blood of normal individuals under the age of twenty-five and the *rise* of cholesterol in the blood of atherosclerotic individuals, Dr. Spittle says. The *fall* in cholesterol in the under-twenty-five age group, she suggests, might have been brought about because the ascorbic acid in essence made it easier for the body to break down cholesterol before it had a chance to become a problem in key areas like arteries. The *rise* in cholesterol levels of patients with atherosclerosis, she added, may have come about because ascorbic acid may have helped chase cholesterol out of the arteries.[1] Atherosclerosis, she concludes, is caused by a long-term deficiency (or even a negative balance) of ascorbic acid, which allows cholesterol levels to build up within the arteries. Moreover, Dr. Spittle says, since ascorbic acid provides material for a sound and healthy ground substance for arterial walls, a lack of vitamin C could, in addition, lead to structurally weak arterial walls, prone to infestation by atherosclerotic-inducing materials. Everyone, she concludes, could have good clean, fat-free arteries simply by eating fruits and vegetables and by eating them fresh. "It was not intended that we should cook, can, or desiccate our fruits and vegetables," she wrote to *Lancet*. "We were expected to eat them raw. Thus the lowest incidence of deaths from coronary thrombosis would be expected at the end of the summer period, after we have spent several months eating these foods. The highest incidence would be expected in early spring, after a few months of cooking them to a degree that renders them useless. . . .[2]

"If the public can produce this striking drop in their death rate without making a conscious effort, how much greater will the fall in the death rate be if they are told what to do. *Please* tell them to eat other fruits and vegetables raw!"

Other researchers have different views of ascorbic acid's role in cholesterol levels. Some of the studies highly touted by those who see ascorbic acid as a new drug against cholesterol, atherosclerosis, and heart disease, critics say, were carried out in dubious fashion. One ascorbic-acid enthusiast, for example, published the results of an intricate study in which heart-disease patients with high cholesterol levels showed marked improvement when ascorbic acid in high doses was added to their diets. What this researcher somehow

---

[1] This warrants an explanation: blood samples are normally taken from the veins. Thus, in Spittle's eyes, an increase in vein serum cholesterol could indicate a fall in arterial cholesterol—and it is in the arteries, after all, where saturated fats cause their greatest damage.

[2] See Introduction.

overlooked, critics say, is that he had also placed his experiment subjects on a very strict fat-free diet. Why he attributed the dramatic improvement in cholesterol levels to ascorbic acid and not to the fat-free diet escapes most atherosclerosis researchers.

Perhaps a vitamin C deficiency may lead to an increase in cholesterol levels, some critics say. However, they add, that does not prove that cholesterol levels will be influenced in any way when high doses of vitamin C are given to people whose tissues are already saturated with the vitamin. Some researchers have reported that giving 1 to 6 grams of ascorbic acid to high-cholesterol patients for six to sixteen weeks had absolutely no therapeutic effect on their cholesterol levels. Dr. T. W. Anderson, of the School of Hygiene at the University of Toronto, found that, contrary to Dr. Spittle's reports, ascorbic acid does not lower cholesterol levels in young adults. Dr. Anderson, who conducted a large double-blind study of ascorbic acid's effectiveness in treating the common cold (see pages 159–161), drew two blood samples from forty-one of his younger (between the ages of eighteen and twenty-four) cold-study subjects. One blood sample was drawn during the last ten days of his study and one six weeks after the study had been completed and high ascorbic-acid levels had been allowed to fall back to normal. Eighteen of the young people had been on vitamin C. Twenty-three had been on a placebo. "Contrary to the hypothesis being tested [that ascorbic acid lowers cholesterol in young people]," Anderson reported in *Lancet,* "not only was the mean serum-cholesterol of the vitamin group higher than that of the placebo group during the last ten days of the trial (194 compared with 185 mg per 100 ml), but there was no evidence of a return to higher cholesterol levels following discontinuation of the large vitamin-C intake (the mean serum-cholesterol of the post-trial samples was 193 and 185 per 100 ml respectively)."

Some doctors even worry that perhaps Dr. Spittle—and others—are right when they say that they detect a rise in serum cholesterol levels in older people given high doses of vitamin C: the rise is there, all right, they say, but it may mean trouble. The serum cholesterol rise, Dr. R. J. Morin of Harbor General Hospital, a UCLA-affiliated hospital in Torrance, California, suggests, might come about because vitamin C sets in motion some mechanisms that lead the body to produce more cholesterol and inhibits others that might be involved in helping the body excrete cholesterol from the body. Ascorbic acid might also force cholesterol out of other tissues where it had been safely tucked away. In other words, ascorbic acid might do everything *but* flush cholesterol out of the arteries. "The rise in serum-cholesterol levels produced in atherosclerotic patients by large doses of vitamin C may actually aggravate the existing atherosclerosis, and the indiscriminate use of these doses for possible prevention of upper respiratory infections and other ailments should be discouraged until the mechanisms of this hypercholesterolaemic effect and other possible toxic effects are fully explored," Dr. Morin suggests.

In 1979, a Houston researcher, Dr. William Hermann, added a new twist to the debate by announcing that vitamin E could influence the levels of the various lipoproteins in the blood. Lipoproteins, the compounds that carry various fatty substances, including cholesterol, are themselves divided into various categories. The most important among them are the high-density lipoproteins (HDL) and the low-density lipoproteins (LDL). Within the last few years, moreover, researchers have found that people who have a high HDL/LDL ratio—that is, more high-density lipoproteins in relation to the number of low-density lipoproteins—have a significantly lower risk of having a heart attack than people with lower HDL/LDL ratios.

According to Hermann's first reports, patients who were given vitamin E had a significant increase in their HDL, thus raising the crucial ratio. When other researchers were unable to confirm the link between vitamin E and increases in HDL, Dr. Hermann reexamined his position. His new conclusion was that the differences in HDL among the men he studied could be more accurately attributed to the ages of the men and their HDL levels before they were given vitamin E than to the vitamin itself.

The debates over vitamin C's alleged effectiveness in curing an assorted number of ills (not as many as E, but quite a few, anyway) ranging from atherosclerosis to slipped discs has involved many doctors and vitamin advocates. But while these debates have sparked some interesting fires, they really have been only sideshows, preliminary bouts to the real debate, the real war involving vitamin C—the war fought over its effectiveness as an anti-cold compound.

CHAPTER VIII

Vitamin C vs. the Common Cold

At one time or another in its long, illustrious career as the public's favorite on the vitamin shelf, ascorbic acid has been put forth as an effective bulwark against dental disease, tuberculosis, bleeding ulcers, lead poisoning, back problems, atherosclerosis, whooping cough, diphtheria, typhoid fever, and mental and emotional problems. Many of the proposed medical uses for vitamin C have been ignored by mainstream doctors, have been proven to be of little substance, or have just been abandoned at the wayside as vitamin enthusiasts have gone on to other interests. But one claim—that ascorbic acid, taken in high doses, can prevent and ameliorate the common cold—has survived for better than thirty years, engaging scientists, doctors, and the lay public in a sometimes low-simmering, sometimes vitriolic, but apparently never-ending debate.

In fairness to other vitamins and their advocates, it must be said that vitamin C is not the first vitamin to be presented as an effective anti-common-cold vitamin. In the 1930s, vitamin A, vitamin A combined with D in cod-liver oil, and vitamin preparations that included A, B_1, B_2, and D were recommended as powerful common-cold preventatives and common cold cures. But the campaigns for these other pretenders to the public's trust and affection never really gained momentum.

In part, these other vitamins failed to gain acceptance as anti-cold remedies because there were never any impressive studies to bear out the claims made in their behalf as anti-cold weapons. Nor did an eminent scientific personality ever indicate a willingness to bear the vitamins' standards. These other vitamins may also have failed because they were often prescribed in foul-tasting preparations that had to be swallowed to reap the alleged anti-cold benefits. More often than not, A and D were prescribed in the form of cod-liver oil, a preparation no one in his right mind would take joyously. It was all right to force the stuff down the throats of children—who could not put up too much of a fight—to help them grow up healthy and strong. But one suspects that even if a score of studies acceptable to the scientific community had confirmed the value of A and D in fighting colds, they would not—not as long as they were dissolved in cod-liver oil—have gained wide acceptance among adults.

Vitamin C, though, is different. The vitamin is available in things—oranges, orange juice, other fruits—the public can actually like. High dosages have been available in simple pills for a long time. Ascorbic acid proved its value (albeit in another disease) in dramatic fashion—it cured the scurvy. It cured the infections that accompanied scurvy. It was, therefore, not hard to imagine that, even in the absence of scurvy, ascorbic acid might cure other infections—like the common cold. Finally, the continuing fascination with ascorbic acid's anti-cold properties can be traced to yet an additional factor: a long string of studies, some well conducted, others badly carried out, that have yielded not only contradictory results but results interpreted in contradictory fashion by both sides to the vitamin-C-common-cold debate; studies, in short, that have kept the debate alive and well.

In 1937 two University of Edinburgh researchers, A. J. Glazebrook and Scott Thompson, undertook a study of vitamin C's effectiveness against some common infections, particularly colds. They conducted their study at a large school in Great Britain where boys from lower socioeconomic strata came to learn a trade. The boys not only attended classes at the school but also lived there. According to Glazebrook and Thompson, the conditions for establishing whether or not supplemental doses of vitamin C are effective against common infections were just right at the school because the boys had to live on what had to be considered nutritionally bad food. ''The food distribution was badly managed,'' Glazebrook and

Thompson reported. "Electric ovens were used to reheat the food, and to keep it hot whilst awaiting distribution. Often 8 hr [*sic*] elapsed between the time the food was cooked and its arrival on the dining tables. The minimum time that heat was applied to food, including the original cooking and the subsequent reheating was 2 hr." All this cooking, heating, reheating, and long periods of storage virtually ensured that the vitamin C content of the diet was uniformly poor. Twelve ounces of potatoes—the amount allotted to each boy—the two researchers said, should have contained at least 50 milligrams of ascorbic acid. By the time the potatoes reached the boys, they contained an average of only 4 milligrams of ascorbic acid. Other foods were similarly depleted, and the total intake of vitamin C averaged barely 10 to 15 milligrams a day for each youngster, just enough to stave off scurvy.

The boys were divided into various groups. In some groups, the boys received high doses of vitamin C (without their knowledge: the ascorbic acid was added in powder form to the cocoa they received in the morning and to the milk they drank at night) until they began to excrete high amounts of vitamin C, indicating that their tissues were now saturated with ascorbic acid and that the body was ridding itself of what it could not use or store. When the levels of saturation had been reached, the amount of supplemental vitamin C given to those boys chosen to receive the vitamin was cut back to 50 milligrams a day, enough to keep each boy at the saturation level.

The study, Glazebrook and Thompson reported, yielded one result favorable to vitamin C (a result they passed on without comment): while there had been seventeen cases of pneumonia and sixteen cases of acute rheumatism among the boys who had continued eating their normal diets without receiving any additional vitamin C, there had been no cases of either illness among the boys who had been given vitamin C. The odds that this would happen by chance, the researchers pointed out, are only one in fifty. Despite this finding, the two researchers could find no reason to get excited about vitamin C's potential as a fighter against infectious disease. Of the boys who received ascorbic acid, 21.2 percent came down with colds. Of the boys who had received no additional vitamin C, 26 percent suffered from colds during the experiment—not a significantly higher number, the researchers pointed out. Nor were there any differences in the incidence of tonsillitis: of those boys given vitamin C, 8.5 percent had tonsillitis. Of those given no C, 8.6 percent suffered from bouts with the disease. The only possible advantage to vitamin C supplementation seemed to be that it resulted in fewer days of illness among the boys who did come down with tonsillitis. But, Glazebrook and Thompson went on to point out, "no such difference was found in the cases of the common cold."

In the same year that Glazebrook and Thompson published the results of their study, three University of Minnesota researchers reported on a study they had conducted with vitamin C among college students.

As the school year began at the university in 1939, the three researchers, Dr. Donald W. Cowan, Dr. Harold S. Diehl, and Dr. A. B. Baker, asked students who thought they were highly susceptible to colds to volunteer for a study at the university's "Cold Prevention Group"; 427 students answered the call. Of the total, 183 were given 200 milligrams of ascorbic acid a day for twenty-eight weeks—the so-called common-cold season in the northern state. Another 50 students were also given ascorbic acid but were instructed to vary their intake of the vitamin: they were to take 200 milligrams a day for the first two weeks, then 100 milligrams a day as long as they felt healthy. If they felt a cold coming on, they were to up their vitamin C intake to 500 milligrams a day for two days and then drop back to 100 milligrams a day. The other students—194 in number—were given a placebo that looked and tasted like ascorbic acid. They were told to take two of these pills, which as far as they knew contained an active drug—twice a day for the same twenty-eight weeks.

The results, Cowan, Diehl, and Baker reported, were not very favorable, as far as they were concerned, to vitamin C. Before the study had begun, each student had supplied a medical history, including an estimate of the number of colds he had suffered the previous year. The students who had been taking vitamin C, analysis of the data revealed, had suffered 5.5 colds a person the year before the study but had suffered only 1.9 colds while they were on vitamin C. The students in the placebo group had suffered an average of 5.9 colds the previous year—but under the placebo they had suffered only 2.2 colds. It was true, the researchers said, that the drop in colds had been greater among the vitamin C group than among the placebo group (the 1.9 colds among the vitamin C students represented a 65.5 percent drop from the previous year, whereas the 2.2 colds among the placebo group represented only a 62.7 drop in colds as compared to the previous year). "Vitamin C supplement to the diet may therefore be judged to give a slight advantage in reducing the number of colds experienced," the trio concluded. "However, one may well question the practical importance of such a [slight] difference."

Neither the Glazebrook and Thompson study nor the University of Minnesota study laid the ascorbic-acid issue to rest. In 1959, a German researcher reported that he had given two thousand factory workers either a placebo or ascorbic acid (in 100- to 300-milligram doses every day) for eight months and that those workers who had been given the supplemental ascorbic acid had been ill far less frequently than those given the placebo. In 1956, three other researchers reported that they had given forty-four medical students and nursing students some 200 milligrams of ascorbic acid a day for three months and that they had compared the incidence of colds among them with a group of forty-five medical students and student nurses who had not gotten vitamin C supplements. Both groups, the researchers said, had virtually the same number of colds. But the group receiving the vitamin C, they said, had less severe colds and had them for a fewer number of days than the students who had received no C.

High school basketball players—boys and girls—who took vitamin preparations that included 200 milligrams of ascorbic acid, a North Carolina physician, Frank E. Barnes, reported in 1961, suffered fewer colds and were generally healthier than students who received no vitamin supplements. The physician had prescribed vitamin supplements for twenty-six basketball players. Twelve girl basketball players had 19 days of colds and five days of flu, Dr. Barnes reported. Only two girls out of the twelve lost time in school in order to stay home to nurse their illnesses. The boy basketball players had 16 days of colds, and they also lost only 2 days of schooling. On the other hand, Dr. Barnes said, the sixteen boys and girls who were not basketball players, and who did not receive vitamin supplements, had 110 days of colds among them during the same period. "The coaches and school officials noted a definite   improvement   in   the   students   given   the   vitamin supplementation, both in their attitudes and playing abilities, from that observed in previous years when no supplements had been given,'' Dr. Barnes reported. ''The coaches were enthusiastic about the greatly reduced number of absences from practice and games.''

In 1961 Dr. G. Ritzel, a physician with the school system in Basel, Switzerland, reported that a study he had carried out with teen-age boys attending ski camps in the Alps had yielded proof that vitamin C could have a positive effect on colds. Ritzel had included 279 boys in his study. He gave 139 of them 1,000 milligrams of vitamin C a day and he gave 140 boys an inert placebo. To make sure that the physicians who were helping in the study would not let their assessment of the experiment be influenced by their prejudices for or against vitamin C, the study was conducted double-blind. The physicians who were asked to assess the health of the boys did not know which boys were receiving the placebo and which were receiving the ascorbic acid. The 139 boys who had been given ascorbic acid, Dr. Ritzel reported, had caught only seventeen colds while they were skiing. The 140 students who had received the placebo had caught thirty-one colds during their week on the slopes.

In 1968 another physician, Dr. Edme Regnier, reported in the *Review of Allergy* that, as far as he was concerned, vitamin C is the answer to the common cold. Dr. Regnier undertook a study of the effect of high doses of vitamin C on twenty-two people who had, in years past, averaged about three colds a year. Each participant in the study was asked to take a dose of 600 or 625 milligrams of C every three hours within the first twenty-four hours of a cold, 375 to 400 milligrams every three hours for the next two or three days, and then about 200 to 250 milligrams every three to six hours until it was evident that the cold had subsided. ''In this small group of subjects,'' Dr. Regnier reported, ''there was not one who failed to obtain successful results as regards his symptomatic response if his intake of ascorbic acid was both sufficient and well timed. . . . As far as the subjects themselves were concerned there was no question on this point because the suppression of the symptoms was so gratifying.''

Proper use of vitamin C, Dr. Regnier continued, would also prevent the onset of colds. ''From observations made over a span of a number of years it appears to me that when one is exposed to an obvious source of infection, as when a patient sneezes in one's face, a dose of 600–750 mg of vitamin C will prevent a possible cold, especially when a second dose of the same magnitude is taken three hours later," Dr. Regnier said. ". . . Before going to the theater where one may be exposed to many people suffering from colds, a prophylactic dose may be taken before leaving home and another 750 mg dose upon returning, with gratifying absence of the usual possible infections."

The enthusiastic reports about ascorbic acid's effectiveness against the cold did not go completely unchallenged, of course.

One group of researchers reported that 147 volunteers who took 3,000 milligrams of vitamin C as soon as they felt a cold coming on and who continued on the high-ascorbic-acid dosage until the colds disappeared—in some cases, fourteen days later—fared no better than another group of 123 volunteers who were given a placebo to "treat" an incipient cold. According to the researchers, they could detect no differences between the groups in either the severity or duration of the colds.

An English group from the Common Cold Research Unit in Salisbury, England (a group that has been studying the common cold for more than thirty years), also reported negative studies involving ascorbic acid.

The researchers, Georgina H. Walker, M. L. Bynoe, and A. J. Tyrell, conducted a three-part study. First they saturated various tissues taken from human lungs and monkey kidneys and cultured them in test tubes, with high doses of ascorbic acid. Then they exposed the tissues to various viruses that cause common colds in human beings. The cultured tissues, the Walker group said, did not prove to be any more resistant to the viruses than tissues not treated with ascorbic acid. The researchers then treated live mice with high doses of ascorbic acid and then exposed them to one flu virus. These mice proved to be no less susceptible to the virus than mice not treated with ascorbic acid.

Finally the Walker group turned to human volunteers. They divided ninety-one human volunteers into two groups. One group of forty-seven persons was given 3 grams of ascorbic acid for three days. The other forty-four volunteers were given a placebo. Both groups were then exposed to common-cold viruses (the researchers sprayed high concentrations of the viruses into the noses and throats of the volunteers). Eighteen of the forty-seven ascorbic-acid volunteers and eighteen of the forty-four placebo volunteers developed colds—a slight difference of about 6 percent. Thirteen of the ascorbic-acid volunteers developed sore throats, as did fifteen of the placebo takers. "We conclude," the researchers reported, "that there is no evidence that the administration of ascorbic acid has any value in the prevention or treatment of colds produced by five known viruses."

For almost thirty years the debate over the effectiveness of ascorbic acid was conducted along fairly civilized, polite lines. Those who did not believe in ascorbic acid pointed out that trials with the vitamin and placebos proved once more that for some strange reason any regimen or therapy could be effective against the disease. "Our studies show that placebos frequently give what appear to be excellent results," Dr. Diehl told a panel discussing ascorbic acid. "It is common for the control group to report a reduction from an average of five to about two colds a year. In fact, certain results reported by many persons who received placebos would serve as splendid testimonials for anything for the preventions of colds." That anything—even injections of sterile water—can lead to a 65 percent decrease in colds, Dr. Cowan said, might have one explanation: "When one is taking two or three pills every day or is given a shot in the arm once or twice a week because he is cold susceptible he is continually being reminded that he is trying to do something about his colds; and he might consciously or unconsciously practice better general hygiene. For example, at Minnesota students are often observed dashing from their rooming houses to the corner drug store at 20 below zero without hats or coats. I wonder whether they aren't more likely to put on a hat and coat when they are in the cold prevention group."

The positive ascorbic-acid studies, the critics said in a low tone of voice, also left a good deal to be desired. The Barnes study in North Carolina, some said, could not be taken seriously because the group given ascorbic acid was composed of youngsters who in all probability took good care of themselves anyway. They considered themselves sportsmen and -women and adhered to a better regimen of self-care than other youngsters. The basketball players probably ate better, got more rest, and certainly exercised more than non-playing youngsters, in order to stay in training. That in itself probably strengthened their resistance to colds. The Ritzel study, others pointed out, clearing their throats politely, just wasn't all that conclusive. The statistical difference between the ascorbic-acid-filled skiers and the placebo-filled skiers was not statistically significant. In any case, someone said, anyone conducting a study with a bunch of kids on a one-week skiing holiday would have to expect that any youngster would downgrade an incipient cold anyway, fearing that he would be kept off the slopes if he gave even the slightest indication that he felt ill.

Those who believed in ascorbic acid quietly demurred. The critics, they said, were either blinding themselves to convincing statistics that ascorbic acid would help or were themselves relying on questionable studies. How could anyone, they asked, take the Walker experiment seriously? People catch colds by being exposed to some viruses floating about in the air around them and the amount of ascorbic acid suggested—three grams or so a day—is probably good enough to take on the common colds engendered by viruses that reach the human organism in so diffuse a fashion. But the Walker group, it was pointed out, sprayed huge concentrations of viruses directly into people, and it was very possible that a mere three grams of ascorbic acid would not be effective against so massive an invasion of cold-causing viruses.

All this well-modulated scientific chitchat ceased suddenly in 1970. In that year Linus Pauling published his *Vitamin C and the Common Cold* and for the second time in almost as many years threw the scientific and medical communities into paroxysms of rage.

After Irwin Stone, the chemist he met at dinner, wrote and suggested he take a high-vitamin-C regimen to help him stay healthy and to help him live longer, Professor Pauling wrote in his 109-page book, he and his wife began to take ascorbic acid in high doses. "We noticed an increased feeling of well-being, and especially, a striking decrease in the number of colds and their severity," Pauling said. Struck by the gratifying results, he added, he began to sift through the common-cold-ascorbic-acid literature. He found that in previous years many of his fellow scientists had ignored the value of high doses of ascorbic acid because they had, in effect, been approaching the whole subject of vitamin C with tunnel vision.

Most scientists, Pauling said, had ignored valuable information that a handful of more imaginative researchers had developed. In 1949 Dr. Geoffrey Bourne had speculated that man's ascorbic-acid requirements might be much higher than just a few milligrams of the stuff a day. "Man's nearest zoological relations are the great apes," Dr. Bourne had told a meeting of the British Nutrition Society in 1949. "The gorilla weighs more than a man and its average energy requirement is probably something like 4,000 to 5,000 kilocalories per day. The chief food of these creatures in the wild is grass or leaves, which have a low energy value. In fact, to obtain 4,000 calories, it would be necessary for a gorilla to eat at least 20 pounds of greenstuff a day. Twenty pounds of such green feed would provide about 4.5 grams of vitamin C daily. Before the development of agriculture and large-scale growing of cereals which made the development of civilization possible, it is likely that man existed largely on greenstuff supplemented with what meat on the hoof he could catch. It may be possible that when we are arguing whether 7 or 30 milligrams is an adequate intake we may be very wide off the mark. Perhaps we should be arguing whether one or two grams a day is the correct amount." Dr. Pauling accepted Bourne's argument. But he extended it by adding that he himself had checked the vitamin C content of some 110 foods, including 14 plants richest in vitamin C that might have been eaten by early man. As a result, Pauling said, he believes that the "optimum daily intake of ascorbic acid for most adult human beings lies in the range 2.3g to 9g."

Pauling's conclusion that man's requirement for vitamin C is actually spread over a broad range is based in part on the theories presented by another researcher he considers to be more imaginative than most other scientists and nutritionists, Professor Roger Williams of the University of Texas at Austin. Williams, Pauling said, has been pointing out for a long time that there is no such thing as an "average" human being, that everyone has different nutritional and biochemical needs. In fact, Pauling wrote, Williams and a colleague, Gary Deason, had carried out a significant experiment with guinea pigs which had demonstrated that not all members of the same species have exactly the same requirements for nutrients.

In a paper read before the National Academy of Sciences, Williams and Deason had reported that they had divided 102 baby guinea pigs into eight different groups. Each group was fed basically the same diet—only the amounts of ascorbic acid were varied from group to group. "The results," Williams and Deason told the gathered members of the academy, "were almost incredibly striking. Each one of the animals exhibited enhanced growth when the high level of intake was further increased. . . . It becomes impossible to escape the conclusion that levels of vitamin C much higher than heretofore reported are needed by *some guinea pigs* for continued growth and maximum growth." One animal received no vitamin C. Like other animals in its subgroup who were also completely deprived of C, this one guinea pig developed scurvy. But unlike the other subgroup members, which had died as a result of their disease, the one guinea pig lived and maintained its weight during the length of the experiment. Two other animals that were put on a low-vitamin-C ration gained weight on their deprived diet. One of them actually grew larger than a number of other animals that were getting two to sixteen times as much ascorbic acid as it was. "We can only conclude," Williams and Deason told the academy, "that at least a 20-fold range in the vitamin C needs of individual guinea pigs exists. . . . On unemotional, scientific grounds it would appear that interindividual variation in human vitamin C needs is probably just as great." Pauling concurred. He wrote that he had "accepted their conclusions and similar conclusions reached by other investigators. . . ."

His fellow scientists, Pauling also said, had erroneously denied the validity of some very convincing experiments that had borne out the value of ascorbic acid in the treatment of the common cold. Worse, said Pauling, even scientists whose experiments had yielded obviously encouraging results had insisted on misinterpreting their own data. Cowan, Diehl, and Baker, Pauling said, had concluded that roughly 200 milligrams of vitamin C given daily had no effect on the common cold, brushing aside the fact that the difference between the students who had taken ascorbic acid and those who had taken a placebo was one third of a cold. This seemingly insignificant reduction, Pauling said, could be extrapolated into "a decrease in the number of colds during the winter by 15 percent. . . . I think that such a difference does have practical importance. Also, the investigators might have asked whether taking twice as much ascorbic acid, 400 milligrams per day, would have decreased the number of colds by twice as much, 30 percent.''

The Cowan study, Pauling said, had yielded additional evidence in ascorbic acid's behalf: although 20 percent of the students given placebos dropped out of the study before the experiment had finished, only 10 percent of the students who were getting the ascorbic acid ended their participation in the study. The obvious conclusion, Pauling said, was that the students in the ascorbic-acid group felt that they were receiving some benefit from the treatment with ascorbic acid—otherwise more would have dropped out. Finally, Pauling said, the students receiving the placebo lost an average of 1.6 days of school, whereas the ascorbic-acid group lost only 1.1 days—a 30 percent differential. Deciphering the results of the Glazebrook and Thompson experiment for himself, Pauling said that the incidence of colds was 13 percent lower among the training students receiving ascorbic acid than among those receiving no supplementation. The Cowan study, the Glazebrook study, the Ritzel and Regnier observations, a host of other experiments, Pauling said, convinced him that ascorbic acid's effectiveness against colds was everything a few daring researchers had said it was.

There was nothing essentially new, then, in what Professor Pauling had said. Nevertheless, the greater part of the scientific and medical community reacted (and still is reacting) as if Pauling had suggested a return to leeching. One medical journal pointed out that Pauling's publisher, W. H. Freeman, was intimately involved in the manufacture and sale of ascorbic acid—an inaccurate statement that the journal was quickly forced to retract. In the fury that followed the publication of the book, the magazine *Science* refused to publish one of Pauling's articles on ascorbic acid. But *Science* was not the only publication to react boorishly, to arbitrarily impose censorship on the theories of a man generally hailed as an important scientist. For almost the entire span of its existence, the highly prestigious National Academy of Sciences—of which Pauling is a member—has accepted for automatic publication in its journal articles submitted by members (articles submitted to most scientific journals of any repute are reviewed and passed upon by an editorial board). But when Professor Pauling submitted an article on ascorbic acid, the editorial board of the *Proceedings of the National Academy of Sciences* refused to publish the piece—the first time in fifty-seven years it had refused to print an article by a NAS member. Even the NAS was embarrassed by the action. Ultimately it apologized to Professor Pauling.

Pauling's book, too, came under scathing attack. Commissioner Charles C. Edwards, the head of the Food and Drug Administration, said the popularity of Pauling's book was "ridiculous." "The many admirers of Linus Pauling will wish that he had not written this book," one reviewer wrote. "Here are found, not the guarded statements of a philosopher or scientist seeking truth, but the clear, incisive sentences of an advertiser with something to sell. . . ." Scientists, doctors, nutritionists reacted with almost unprecedented venom. "Dr. Pauling's positions on vitamin C . . . are an embarrassment for an older scientist," Dr. George E. Moore, director of surgical oncology in the Denver Department of Health and Hospitals, said. "This episode is not the first time a great scientist has been wrong. Look at Krebiozen,[1] where an important investigator went gung-ho. Creative men have been known to perpetrate bummers. This may be one of those occasions." "This is the second nutritional fairy tale (the first was 'Orthomolecular Psychiatry') to come from this intelligent and likable man," Doctors Frederick J. Stare and K. C. Hayes of the Department of Nutrition at the Harvard School of Public Health said. "Like Hansel and Gretel, he is lost in the woods—of health and nutrition, areas outside his competence."

Nutritionists in particular are livid over Pauling's excursions into the realm they consider their exclusive satrapy. Pauling's contentions that prehistoric or primitive man ingested far greater amounts of ascorbic acid than modern man, these nutritionists say, is utter nonsense. "There is no evidence that there was higher vitamin C intake in the past," Dr. Leo Lutvak says. "As a matter of fact, the evidence is that there was less. Primitive man had no means of food preservation or storage. His vitamin C intake was dependent on the seasons. There were certain periods of the year

---

[1] Moore was probably referring to Dr. Andrew C. Ivy. Ivy, a prominent physiologist, author of fifteen hundred papers in his field and winner of four American Medical Association research medals, became a staunch believer in Krebiozen, a highly controversial anti-cancer "drug." Although the "drug," made from a horse-serum derivative, never gained acceptance in medical circles because its worthiness went largely unproven, Ivy continued to believe and fight for it, even though his stance eventually cost him his job as a vice-president of the University of Illinois.

when he would have fresh fruit available for a few weeks, but the rest of the time, he wouldn't have any. He might have taken grams of C at a time, for one or two days of the year, but since C is not stored it would have all been excreted anyway.''

He has checked Dr. Pauling's list of high-ascorbic-acid foods available to modern man's distant ancestors, Professor Thomas Jukes says, and found it wanting. ''Primitive man did not have the plants that give Pauling his high figures,'' Professor Jukes says. ''Cauliflower, brussels sprouts, broccoli spears, black currants, hot chili peppers are products of horticulture. All right, berries are very high. Yes. But it is more likely that primitive men relied more on nuts and grains as a source of food because they were the ones they could store through the winter.

''There is no test that shows that man needs that much vitamin C. If he did, he would never have been able to spread all over the world. He suffered scurvy because he got less than 10 milligrams of C. But two grams? If he had needed that much C, he would have never gotten out of the tropics. If we had needed such a high level of C, we would never have given up the genetic machinery to make it. There is no benefit in giving it up because all other animals, except the great apes and the guinea pig, have it, and there is no logic at all in the way the ascorbic acid synthesizing machinery is distributed in the animal kingdom. The myna bird, which can make C, subsists on berries. Swallows, which cannot make C, eat insects, which are low in C. There is no logic in it all.''

There is probably little harm in Pauling's discussions and theories of the evolution of man's ascorbic-acid needs, many nutritionists and scientists feel. But there is a great deal of harm in his foray into a branch of science he does not really understand—applied medicine. It is one thing, they say, to sit in a laboratory and spin theoretical webs about the origins and treatment of a disease. It is quite another to deal face to face with some of these problems, to try to understand the very subtle effects of medical treatment of some human ills. That Pauling is a Nobel laureate in Chemistry, Dr. Jean Mayer, Harvard's popular nutritionist, wrote in *Family Health,* ''does not invalidate Will Rogers' wise maxim that 'we are all ignorant about different things.' In Professor Pauling's case, the weak spot seems to be epidemiology, the difficult discipline that deals with the evaluation of medical statistics—a far cry from organic chemistry.'' Pauling, in other words, might be able to calculate with exquisite precision whether or not the number of times a specific reaction in a test tube is statistically significant, whether or not the number of times the reaction takes place bears out the experimenter's theorems. But knowing how to deal with statistics in the chemistry laboratory, the critics say, does not give him the insight to evaluate statistics derived from experiments undertaken in a field other than his own.

Pauling dismisses the criticisms. ''I have tried to understand why physicians, nutritionists, authorities and even investigators have done the things they have done,'' he says. ''It is hard to understand physicians, I must say. They believe in authoritarianism and they apparently find it hard to understand that the world changes. They form their beliefs early, perhaps when they are in medical school. They accept what they are told. I think it is good for a physician to be conservative. But they seem to me to be too unwilling to consider anything different.''

During his fight to have vitamin C recognized as the one and only effective compound capable of defeating the common cold, Pauling has had few defenders within what might be called the establishment circles of medicine and science. *Hospital Tribune,* a newspaper distributed to physicians in hospitals, gave Pauling a long, sympathetic airing by running series of question-and-answer articles in which Pauling was allowed to put forth—virtually without challenge—all his ideas and theories. ''As the controversy [over vitamin C] continued,'' *Hospital Tribune* said in its introduction to its presentation of Pauling's views, ''a tendency to attack Dr. Pauling in an obscure, insinuating way developed. Were they motivated by his opposition to the war in Vietnam, by his criticism of the medical profession, or by his criticism of FDA-approved cold remedies? . . . Did physicians feel threatened by the fact that the public was reading this book?''

That *Hospital Tribune,* not *Science* or the *Proceedings of the National Academy of Sciences,* should allow Pauling the privilege of presenting his point of view is not without irony. Pauling's book contains a chapter scoring unmercifully the dangers of conventional drugs available to control the symptoms of colds. He also cites, with apparent approval, the comments of a doctor who wrote in *Fact* magazine that ''having worked as a researcher in the field, it is my contention that effective treatment for the common cold, a cure, is available, that is being ignored because of the monetary losses that would be inflicted on pharmaceutical manufacturers, professional journals, and doctors themselves.'' That cure, the doctor had written, was ascorbic acid. "Dr. Gildersleeve [the author-physician's nom de plume]," Dr. Pauling notes in his own book, "reported . . . that in 1964 he wrote a paper in which he described his observations [about vitamin C]. He submitted the paper to eleven different professional journals, every one of which rejected it. Dr. Gildersleeve also reported . . . that one editor said to him that it would be harmful to the journal to publish a useful treatment for the common cold. He stated that medical journals depend for their existence on the support of their advertisers, and that over twenty-five percent of the advertisements in the journals relate to patented drugs for the alleviation of cold symptoms or for the treatment of complications of colds. . . . I think that this anecdote explains in part the slowness with which the value of ascorbic acid has been recognized by the medical profession. . . .'' *Hospital Tribune,* of course, is dependent on drug advertisements for its existence.

Here and there, on a few occasions, someone has spoken up in favor of Pauling. Albert Szent-Györgyi attended a conference on vitamin C and the common cold at Stanford University and told of his faith in vitamin C. He takes, Szent-Györgyi said, two grams of C a day (plus wheat germ) and no longer has colds. "If the body doesn't get enough ascorbic acid, you don't just get a cold," said Szent-Györgyi, now in his eighties and still head of the Institute for Muscle Research at Woods Hole, Massachusetts. "Every-thing—just everything—goes to pieces, and the final stage is scurvy." Szent-Györgyi urged that more studies be undertaken to test Pauling's theory. "There are too few double-blind studies and too many double-blind doctors," he sternly warned. "Dr. Pauling estimated colds cost us $15 billion a year, and the combined ignorance of politicians and physicians keeps us from spending even $1 million a year to prevent them." Pauling has even received a measure of support from one member of the American Medical Association's Council on Food and Nutrition, Dr. Charles E. Butterworth. "It is all too easy," Dr. Butterworth, who is also professor of medicine at the University of Alabama, said, "to withdraw behind a facade of complacency and omniscience. It takes courage, on the other hand, to accept Pauling's challenges and look beyond one's personal involvement and commitments. I suspect that Pauling has done better in his foray into the field of nutrition than most nutritionists could have done in, say, physical chemistry.

"I feel strongly that it would be a terrible mistake if the 'nutrition community' reacted negatively to this book, when a positive, constructive response would be equally justifiable.

"One is haunted by the specter of the British Admiralty waiting 50 years to eliminate scurvy from their Navy—and 100 years to eliminate it from their merchant fleet. It seems to me that this kindly man is chiding the entire medical profession and all nutrition scientists, suggesting that they look to their laurels.''

A few nutrition scientists have taken Dr. Butterworth's advice and have looked "to their laurels." Thus, in the last two or three years, as a handful of research groups have published the results of well-run studies, the tide has shifted somewhat—not greatly, but perceptibly—in Dr. Pauling's favor.

In 1971 Dr. George H. Beaton, head of the nutrition department in the University of Toronto's School of Hygiene, and a colleague reviewed Dr. Pauling's book for the *Canadian Medical Association Journal*. By and large, they didn't look too kindly on the book, scoring its "missionary" writing style, and concluding that Dr. Pauling's claims were "unsubstantiated." However, they added, "when a theoretician as prominent as Linus Pauling puts forth arguments as fervently as he does, unorthodox to the medical scientist as they may be, they warrant consideration. . . . It must be admitted that the opinion of a man who has won two Nobel Prizes must carry some weight even when his remarks apply to a field which differs appreciably from his prime discipline."

Taking his own advice, Dr. Beaton, along with D. B. Reid, and T. W. Anderson, the epidemiologist who has also investigated the claims made for vitamin E, undertook a large-scale study of Dr. Pauling's claims. The researchers began by recruiting one thousand volunteers by combing the School of Hygiene, a local technical school, a local utility company, and a Toronto hospital and by asking everyone interested in their experiment to recruit family, friends, and relatives.

Each volunteer was given a bottle containing 500 tablets. Half of the bottles contained 250-milligram vitamin C pills, half contained a placebo that had been mixed to look and taste like ascorbic acid. To test whether anyone might be able to guess whether he were receiving ascorbic acid or the placebo, the experimenters first asked thirty people to taste both tablets and to try to judge which was ascorbic acid. Sixteen people said the placebo was the ascorbic acid. Fourteen correctly chose the pill actually containing the vitamin C. Thus the researchers were sure that everyone in the experiment thought he was getting ascorbic acid. To ensure that the experimenters themselves would not know who was getting what, each bottle was assigned a code number and the list bearing the code was kept by a statistician who was not part of the research team.

All of the volunteers were given the same instructions: take four pills a day regularly. If you feel a cold coming on, take sixteen pills (4,000 milligrams) the first three days. Each volunteer was given a record sheet that looked like a calendar and was told to note every day whether he felt ill or healthy, and how many tablets he had taken that day. On the other side of the sheet, the volunteers were asked to note, if they had fallen ill, whether they had been mildly, moderately or not at all affected by the illness in such various sites as nose, throat, ears; whether they had suffered from chills; whether they had seen a doctor, stayed away from work or school; whether they had taken some nonprescription drugs. The record sheets were turned in at the end of every month and the information transferred to a computer.

When the study ended nearly four months later, the code was broken and the results analyzed. The researchers, who had admitted right at the start that they were skeptical of Pauling's claims, found that the study had yielded data favorable to vitamin C. There was no significant difference in the average number of colds or the average number of days of sickness in the group that had received the vitamin, the researchers found. "However," they reported, "there was a statistically significant difference between the two groups in the number of subjects who remained free of illness throughout the study period. Furthermore, the subjects receiving the vitamin experienced approximately 30 percent fewer total days of disability (confined to the house or off work) than those receiving the placebo, and this difference was statistically highly significant. The reduction in disability appeared to be due to a lower incidence of constitutional symptoms such as chills, and severe malaise, and was seen in all types of acute illness, including those which did not involve the upper respiratory tract.''

A second study that gave ascorbic acid a sizable boost was conducted by Dr. John L. Coulehan and three associates with schoolchildren enrolled in an elementary school in Steamboat, Arizona.

The children were divided into two groups for the length of the fourteen-week study. One group was given a placebo made to resemble ascorbic acid. The other group received the ascorbic acid itself. Children between the ages of six and ten received one gram of C a day. Children between the ages of ten and fifteen received two grams of C a day. The pills were passed out every day by teachers in the school who made sure that the children actually took their pills and did not hoard or trade them. On weekends or before holidays, the children were given a packet with an appropriate number of pills to be taken under parental supervision. The experimenters, of course, did not know which children were receiving the palcebo, which the ascorbic acid.

When the results of the study were analyzed, it was apparent that ascorbic acid had conferred some special benefit on those children who had been given the vitamin. Both the children given ascorbic acid and the children given the placebo suffered about the same number of colds. However, the children in the group given vitamin C were ill for fewer days than those children on the placebo. Twenty-eight percent of the younger children and 34 percent of the older ones were ill for fewer days than the children on the placebo. The researchers also looked at the other side of the coin. How many children in each group had stayed well during the study? It would have been impossible, of course, to follow each child for fourteen weeks. Thus much of the data for the experiment was gathered on certain ''survey'' days. The researchers found that on these days 32 percent of the children on ascorbic acid had been well (or apparently well), while only 16 percent of the children on the placebo could be said to be free of any illness.

When Coulehan first undertook his experiment, he did so because, among other things, he didn't think that the "absolutely negative reaction to Pauling was warranted because all of the studies had shown some benefits, even if the benefits were limited or small." Nevertheless, Dr. Coulehan added, he and the others were surprised about the results they had obtained in their study with the children at Steamboat.

To be sure that their results were accurate, Coulehan and his associates conducted a second study. In this second trial, some children received vitamin C in 1 gram doses and others received a placebo.

This time around, the group reported, the results yielded by vitamin C were unimpressive. The 133 children taking vitamin C showed 166 cold episodes (that is, upper and lower respiratory tract problems, sore throats, ear infections, and so on) while 129 children on the placebo reported 159 similar episodes of cold related problems. According to the study, there were no significant differences in the number of days the children in each group were absent from school.

Why the difference between the first and the second studies? In essence, the Coulehan group said in the *New England Journal of Medicine,* the positive results that emerged from the first study may have been more a function of the way in which the data were analyzed than of the vitamin itself. In other words, since so many children were involved, since so many different factors were involved—ranging from number of cold "episodes" to days absent—it was plausible that the methods used to make sense out of all the data were primarily responsible for yielding the information that made it seem as if, on a statistical basis, the children who had received vitamin C had been somewhat better off.

The fact that so much statistical study is necessary in itself casts a shadow on the claims for C. If massive doses of ascorbic acid were as powerful and as effective as claimed by Pauling and others, little statistical interpretation would have to be done. The fact that the Coulehan group (as well as other researchers) had to pore over the data in order to discern the difference between the children taking C and the children taking the placebo would make it seem doubtful that vitamin C is worth very much. "It is clear that effects, if any, are . . . modest and inconsistent," the Coulehan group said in summary, adding that all in all vitamin C was not very useful, in their eyes, as a weapon against the cold.

Ultimately, Anderson went on to do additional experiments that tempered somewhat the results of his first study. In essence,

Anderson found that if he gave vitamin C in significantly smaller doses than those suggested by Pauling, these doses too would, once a cold had set in, cut down on the number of days of suffering. In other words, saturating the body's tissues with vitamin C could ameliorate the effects of the cold, but the saturation did not have to be achieved with megadoses of ascorbic acid. "Even in these groups [the subjects who had received lower doses of C and who suffered for fewer days once they came down with colds] there was little or no evidence of an effect on . . . their total duration, or on local [nasal] symptoms," Anderson wrote. "Rather, the effect seemed to be restricted to the severity of the cold as measured by the amount of time spent off work or confined to the house."

What we have left then is this: Taking massive amounts of vitamin C will not guarantee that we will go through life without ever having a cold again, or even reduce the number of colds we do get. But perhaps taking vitamin C in some modest amounts— say 100 to 150 milligrams a day when a cold strikes—may have a small beneficial effect by cutting into the severity of the illness.

The proposition that vitamin C may have a small anti-histaminelike effect on colds once they have started does not, however, close the issue. At least one other question remains: How does vitamin C help ameliorate the effects of a cold?

One school of thought seems to have formed around the proposition that vitamin C's role is marginal. Those who subscribe to this proposition believe C works much like aspirin and a hundred commonly available over-the-counter drugs and compounds. In other words, C may only reduce the inflammations that block noses or trigger coughs. In this view, in other words, vitamin C is only an incidental palliative that does nothing to fight off the agents causing the cold, that does nothing to help the body's immunological system fight off the cold-causing organisms. One study (also cited as proof for the general theorem that vitamin C is effective) conducted in the early 1970s by two Irish researchers established that young girls given 500 milligrams of vitamin C suffered less severe, less intense cold symptoms than girls given a placebo. The researchers, however, on delving deeper into their findings, found that all of the girls getting vitamin C and deriving benefit from it, those girls who had stuffy noses or runny noses were the ones who were getting the greatest benefits from the vitamin. The girls who had more widespread problems—fever, sore throats, headaches—did not seem to fare as well under the vitamin C regimen. According to the Coulehan report in the *New England Journal of Medicine,* the Arizona study yielded much the same results. Children who had coughs or nasal problems had fewers days of illness than children who had also taken vitamin C but who had more generalized cold problems.

These studies, then, seem to indicate that vitamin C has an antihistaminelike effect limited to superficial symptoms.

An opposing school of thought believes that vitamin C might be working at deeper levels, that it works either to destroy viruses, to prevent their spread, or to boost the body's immunological response to colds. Because vitamin C in the Anderson study in Canada seemed to be of help against symptoms that were generalized throughout the body, some observers feel that ascorbic acid does exert its influence through the immunological system. "There is fairly good evidence," Dr. Bourne believes, "that vitamin C has an effect on antibody production. There is also evidence that vitamin C can inactivate some bacterial toxins. Some rather more controversial studies suggest that vitamin C inhibits or slows growth of bacteria. There is also evidence that vitamin C may have an inactivating effect on some viruses."

Anderson, however, seems to doubt that C does its work by taking on bacteria and viruses—though he is willing at least to see that proposition pursued. "Some have suggested that there may be a type of antibiotic effect in which high concentrations of ascorbic acid have a specific antiviral or antibacterial effect," Anderson wrote in *American Pharmacy* in 1979. "Human experiments have not lent much support to this belief, although if it were true, one would expect to see variations in effectiveness depending on the type of virus or bacterium causing the illness, and such variation might help to explain some of the conflicting results obtained in vitamin C trials."

The debate over the true role of vitamin C is of more than just theoretical importance. Right now, if we accept the basic but broad premise that vitamin C is effective against the common cold, we can act on that premise only by gorging ourselves with tens of thousands of grams of ascorbic acid. We would like to believe—some of us fervently so—that something as good, as natural as vitamin C cannot possibly have detrimental effects on the body. But there is, in fact, no rational basis for nurturing this fond wish. The body, in the course of evolution, has become a finely tuned mechanism, and there is nothing, no matter how natural, how seemingly innocuous, that the body can tolerate infinitely in massive doses without suffering damage, damage that is sometimes severe.

Thus, if vitamin C plays no greater role in the body than Contac or Coricidin, if it does nothing but act as a palliative agent to cut down on runny noses, is it worth running the risks of side effects that might be more serious than those engendered by a judicious amount of aspirin (Dr. Pauling's thoughts on the matter notwithstanding) by taking gram after gram of vitamin C (see pages 203-205).

Even if researchers were to find that vitamin C's role is far more important and that it does play a role in the body's immunological resistance to disease, it could be argued that we should delay using it until the specific way in which it acts is worked out. It might very well be that continuing studies will reveal how ascorbic acid in moderate doses could bring about the same effects as Dr. Pauling's megadoses. Research might even reveal that only certain parts of ascorbic acid are active in combating the cold, thus sparing us not just the possible detrimental side effects of vitamin C but also the inconvenience of buying, keeping, and swallowing a heroic and never-ending parade of pills.

CHAPTER IX

Not Letting Facts
Interfere with a Good Story

In the half century or so that has elapsed since it was proposed that chemical compounds called vitamins are responsible for the prevention of certain diseases like scurvy, pellagra, beriberi, and rickets, thousands of researchers have been working fervently—conducting experiments, writing papers, attending an endless number of symposia—to muster some understanding of what these mysterious compounds are really all about.

This monumental effort has allowed science some glimpses into the secrets of vitamins—though not very much. Biochemists and nutritionists obviously know that the lack of vitamins is indeed responsible for some diseases, they know that the vitamins are necessary if the body is to function well. They know that vitamins are important as catalysts for the proper use of food in the body. Aligning themselves with enzymes in the cell, the vitamins act to help the cell convert other nutrients that find their way into the cell into forms of energy the cell can use in its various activities. Furthermore, nutritionists know that foods carry in them the very vitamins that will be needed to metabolize those foods at the cellular level.

Once he has defined that particular role for vitamins, once he has outlined the chemical composition of the vitamins, once he has explained how the vitamins can be synthesized in the laboratory so that they might be mass produced, the "legitimate" vitamin researcher is left hemming and hawing about other aspects of vitamins. The biochemist knows that there are a number of chemical reactions in which ascorbic acid participates. The addition of vitamin C increases somewhat the rates at which those reactions take place. But if vitamin C is not present, the reactions go on anyway. What, then, is the specific role of vitamin C in those reactions? No one knows for sure. The lack of vitamin A leads to serious problems in various tissues in the body—but, again, the vitamin's specific role in maintaining tissue integrity has yet to be identified. Vitamin D, biochemists know, is intimately involved in calcium metabolism. Yet the biochemist who can sketch out on a blackboard in his laboratory vitamin D's exact role in the body's utilization of calcium has yet to make himself known. "We just don't know how vitamins work," Dr. Kaufman of NIH summarizes. "We can describe what they do, but not why they do it."

The large gaps in the knowledge about vitamins, their basic roles, the extent of their actions, have made for the voids that have been so eagerly filled in by doctors and nutritionists who recommend vitamins as effective cures or preventatives for human ills that have otherwise defied conventional medicine. Because much about vitamins is a vast and unexplored terrain, those who believe fervently in vitamins rush in to practice what is known as theoretical medicine, the practice of medicine that says substance X or substance Y works, not because it has been proven beyond a doubt that X or Y are effective, but because theoretically, given a few disparate clues here and there, there is no reason why X or Y should not work in the prescribed fashion.

The process begins more or less this way. The lack of a certain vitamin, vitamin advocates point out, causes a certain deficiency. The deficiency in turn leads to infections, depressions, changes in muscles, changes in the nervous system. The vitamin, given in very modest doses, eradicates the deficiency disease. All the secondary manifestations that were attendant to the deficiency problem also disappear. Conclusion? Massive doses of the vitamins must also be effective against infections, muscle or nerve conditions—anything at all—even if the primary deficiency itself is not present. Somehow, a pound of cure becomes more important than the proverbial ounce of prevention. Similarly, the vitamin advocates point out enthusiastically, vitamin deficiencies in experimental animals lead to diseases similar to those sometimes seen in man. The experimental animal is in no way related to man on the biological scale, nor is the animal version of the disease completely similar to the version seen in man. But that does not matter. Applications of the vitamin cured the disease in the animal. It must also, therefore, be effective in man. "It must be a pleasure," sighs one scientist, surrounded by the paraphernalia of a crowded laboratory, "to be able to leap from point A to point B and think you have a valid conclusion without having to make the necessary fifty intermediary stops between your premise and the conclusion you want to reach."

Vitamin A is a good example of the way theoretical medicine is able to leap over towering diseases in a single bound. Early vitamin researchers found that a vitamin A deficiency was primarily responsible for blinding millions of persons around the world. Without vitamin A, the eye slowly deteriorates. In the early stages of the vitamin deficiency a chemical vital for vision in dim light and for helping the eye adapt to dark is not formed properly—hence the onset of night blindness. As the vitamin deficiency deepens, the cornea of the eye grows soft and the eye tissues themselves start to ulcerate and die. In time, blindness closes in completely.

But researchers also found that, in man as well as animals, vitamin A carries out other important functions. Tooth cells and nervous system cells degenerate if A is not present in sufficient quantities in the diet. Without A, cell division is slowed down, the lining of the respiratory, gastrointestinal, and genitourinary tracts dries out, salivary and endocrine glands dry out. In vitamin-A-deficient animals, the testes are undersized, shrunken, and flabby. Fetuses in vitamin-A-deficient animals show congenital abnormalities, including eye deformities, displaced kidneys, heart abnormalities, growth of extra ears, the appearance of cleft palates and harelips. In many cases, female rats fed vitamin-A-deficient diets abort before delivery. If they carry their young to term, the mothers often die in delivery.

To vitamin enthusiasts, the most important aspect of vitamin A research has been the association found between vitamin A and infections. Research has shown that vitamin A deficiency ultimately leads to the appearance of severe infections in many tissues of the body. Recently, researchers at the National Institute of Allergy and Infectious Diseases fed experimental mice high doses of vitamin A and then injected them with various strains of bacteria. Control mice were also infected with the bacteria but were treated with saline injections. One batch of mice, a group infected with a strain of bacteria known as *Pseudomonas aeroginosa,* reacted spectacularly to the high-vitamin-A doses. Although the mice showed signs of a severe infection during the first three hours following their exposure to the bacteria, by the fifth hour there was no trace at all of the infection in their bloodstreams. All of the non-vitamin-A-treated mice who had been given the same bacterial strain died within twenty-four hours.

All of this has led vitamin advocates to recommend massive doses of vitamin A for a wide variety of human infections, including measles, chicken pox, and scarlet fever. The vitamin, it has been said, would either prevent the diseases or cure them should they have gained a foothold.

But in recommending the use of vitamin A to fight off infections, the vitamin enthusiasts ignore a number of key points in vitamin research. When animals deprived of vitamin A develop infections, the diseases in most instances are highly localized within the body. That is, the infections start and thrive in those areas where tissues, deprived of vitamin A, are breaking down and where dying or dead cells provide excellent breeding ground for bacteria. These are not infections that affect the entire body because a microorganism has gained entry into the bloodstream and is waging war on the entire system. It's the diffference, for example, between an infection in a cut finger and blood poisoning. Researchers have conducted various experiments, furthermore, to show that vitamin A in doses larger than those required to clear up a deficiency and to keep the body well are not useful. Animals deprived of vitamin A, it has been demonstrated, suffer many problems, but they do not lose their ability to produce antibodies, the immunological weapons that fight off diseases. Even the more recent studies at the National Institute of Allergy and Infectious Diseases do not prove very much—except that one strain of mouse, infected by one strain (among thousands) of bacteria, will react favorably when injected with high doses of vitamin A. It is noteworthy that in the experiment all the other mice, treated with other strains of bacteria and injected with vitamin A, died as a result of their infections.

Vitamin enthusiasts also conveniently ignore other data that contradict their views that theoretically vitamin A is a powerful anti-infection agent. When the urine produced by a healthy person is examined, it is found to contain by-products that are formed when vitamin A is broken down and used by the body in the normal course of events. However, analyses of urine produced by people suffering from cancer, tuberculosis, chronic infections, prostate disease, poisonings, and high fever reveal that during these diseases people excrete massive amounts of the vitamin in an unchanged form, indicating that the vitamin, for some unknown reason, is not being broken down and utilized by the body to fight off disease. Perhaps in acute illnesses the body loses its ability to use vitamin A altogether and no amount of the vitamin will do any good anyway. Autopsies of people who have died of infectious diseases have yielded one additional bit of information: virtually without exception, all died with vast supplies of the vitamin still stored in the liver.

When it is pointed out that people who have perfectly normal levels of vitamins in the bloodstream or in the liver (where many vitamins are stored) develop the very diseases the vitamins in massive doses are thought to prevent or cure, the vitamin theoreticians point out that perhaps normal levels or even moderately high levels of a vitamin are not enough. Perhaps, they say, the sufferer of the disease is ill precisely because he is incapable of absorbing or utilizing a particular vitamin at the cellular level where important metabolic activities take place. Perhaps, it is suggested, the bindings that unite vitamins and enzymes within cells into effective metabolic activists are somehow deficient in certain people. Since the metabolic activity is shortcircuited through improper vitamin-enzyme binding, the only way around the difficulty is to bombard the cell with amounts of the vitamin that might be a hundred, or a thousand times bigger than the amounts the body—and the cell— would get under normal circumstances. Under such massive inundation the odds are good, the vitamin practitioners say, that some vitamins will hook onto their enzymatic partners and do the work they are meant to do. Once the metabolic processes are on the right track again, the illness will disappear.

Traditional researchers object to this kind of thinking. There is no doubt that some people do suffer from problems that do not allow them to use vitamins properly. According to the Vitamin Information Bureau, "a patient may suffer malabsorption without knowing it, and some people go around for years without discovering that this is the reason for their day in, day out feeling of sluggishness, lack of energy, and inefficiency." Vitamin malabsorption problems, says the VIB, are "difficult to diagnose and may be taken for all sorts of illnesses, from whooping cough to tuberculosis." However, while this sort of statement is jumped upon with alacrity by vitamin enthusiasts, it is important to look at it in perspective: namely, that the off chance that some of us may have malabsorption problems does not justify scaring millions of people into taking expensive and massive vitamin preparations to protect themselves against a problem they probably do not have. "Maybe one person in 100,000 needs special vitamin therapy because of a metabolic defect," says Dr. Borsook. "But you cannot recommend giving everyone massive doses just to help this rare case. The chances are that if someone thinks he is the one who needs massive doses of vitamins, he is probably a hypochondriac and kidding himself. But if not, he is best off going to a doctor, one well versed in vitamin diseases."

It could be theoretically possible that improper vitamin-enzyme bindings at the cellular level are responsible for faulty metabolic processes within a cell and that illnesses might arise as a result of these malfunctions, biochemists say. And it is also theoretically possible that vitamins administered in huge concentrations might resolve the improper binding difficulties. But another theory—one with somewhat greater support in experiments in bacteria and single-cell organisms—say the doubters, is more likely: namely, that improper vitamin-enzyme bindings are just not the rule in any of the biological processes that mark all life. "You can find tremendous variations in enzyme levels in bacteria," Dr. Kaufman says. "But the situations that would require one hundred times more vitamins haven't occurred. It is unlikely that such a thing is a general phenomenon in nature."

Not even in human beings who are slightly more complex than single-cell bacteria?

"Well, a human being is nothing but billions of bacterial cells all glued together. This has been one of the big discoveries biochemistry has demonstrated in the last ten years of research, that on a cellular level, life is life. Take an elephant, a human being, bacteria. The exact same chemical reactions take place. General metabolic transformations are exactly the same. The same energy-producing reactions that occur in an elephant cell occur in bacterial cells, in plant cells. You can be pretty certain that what you are looking at in microorganisms like *E. Coli* [a bacterium] is also taking place in your next door neighbor." [1]

The problem, of course, is that the two versions of the enzyme-vitamin binding theory are at loggerheads. And, to settle the dispute, some scientist somewhere would have to prove that, in human beings, situations do exist in which there are defective enzyme-vitamin bindings and that massive doses of vitamins will solve the problem. But that is virtually impossible. "To study an enzymatic reaction," says Dr. Kaufman, "you need the enzymes, and they are pretty hard to get. It takes tons of tissue. I need ten kilos of beef liver, fresh, right out of the animal, to get ten milligrams of enzymes. You cannot, in other words, grind up enough people so you can study human enzyme-vitamin bindings."

With virtually no way to resolve the questions about the role of vitamins at the most basic metabolic levels, there is virtually no way to limit the theoretical medicine vitamin enthusiasts would like to practice. In the absence of hard-and-fast knowledge, the vitamin enthusiasts can take any fragment of fact known about a given vitamin and spin a wide and intricate belief about the vitamin's usefulness in, well, anything they want to use the vitamin for. It also means that the vitamin enthusiasts can be very choosy about which facts they will use to support their pet theories.

It is surprising, for example, that no one has yet advocated (as far as I know) the use of massive doses of vitamin B_{12} as a way to prolong life. Nutritionists have found that American blacks have substantially higher levels of B_{12} in their bloodstream than American whites. The life-span of an average black, it is true, is only sixty-two years, while the average life-span of an American white is more or less seventy years. But when black Americans manage to live past the age of sixty-five, they live substantially longer than white Americans who live past sixty-five. Theoretically, it might be

---

[1] Note that Kaufman is talking about very basic chemical reactions. This, however, does not mean that broader systemic activities are necessarily the same.

proposed that B_{12} might be responsible for the increased post-sixty-five longevity in blacks and that everyone should really take massive doses of B_{12}.

While there is no talk of B_{12} as a fountain-of-youth vitamin, there is ample talk about riboflavin as an anticancer vitamin. Many vitamin enthusiasts, choosing their facts very carefully, want to believe, fervently, that a high-vitamin regimen (of riboflavin as well as other vitamins) will protect an individual against cancer and may even cure the dreaded disease if and when it strikes.

The dearth of facts confers an additional benefit on those who believe in the practice of theoretical medicine. It allows them to recommend ingestions of massive doses of vitamins without paying attention to any detrimental effects the high concentrations of the vitamins might have. The theoretical practitioners can ignore the theoretical problems that may come about as a result of their recommendations. They can choose to pay attention only to the "good" facts and to ignore the "bad" facts.

Theoretically, an overabundance of vitamins could cause damage on any number of levels. The vitamin buffs argue that massive doses of vitamins are necessary because metabolic defects could prevent us from utilizing the small amounts of vitamins available to us through our food. But given the wide variability among humans that the vitamin enthusiasts like to assume, it may also be postulated that there are a lot of people whose metabolic processes are overly sensitive to an overabundance of any given vitamin. Researchers have speculated that children with a disease known as Hurler's syndrome suffer from such an oversensitivity, in this case to vitamin C. Vitamin C is important to the formation of connective tissue. Children with Hurler's syndrome suffer from an overproduction of connective tissue, an overproduction that may be behind the grotesque facial features, mental retardation, and eyesight and hearing impairments that are the hallmarks of the disease. Researchers at Stanford University, speculating that an overabundance of C is indeed involved in Hurler's syndrome, placed one baby girl on a completely vitamin-C-free diet. The girl, who was on the diet for over a year, never developed any signs of a vitamin C deficiency, never developed scurvy. Apparently she had been born with a vestigial ability to manufacture vitamin C. That ability, plus the vitamin C she was receiving in the diet, it was speculated, might have caused her problems. Whether a vitamin-C-free diet given early enough would prevent Hurler's syndrome remains to be seen. Nevertheless, it is obvious that, theoretically at least, some people may be harmed by vitamins not just because those vitamins have a deleterious druglike effect but because the body is already using what is available to it all too efficiently and is metabolically incapable of dealing with even the slightest additional amounts of vitamins.

Thus, say many of Pauling's critics, he too ignores other theoretical side effects that could come about as a result of an overly ambitious ingestion of vitamin C. High doses of ascorbic acid, warns Dr. Merton P. Lamden, associate professor of biochemistry at the University of Vermont, have been associated with reproduction problems in guinea pigs. Experimental animals fed vitamin C in high doses conceive less often or yield dead fetuses more often than guinea pigs fed normal amounts of vitamin C. Lamden stresses that there is no evidence that similar problems occur in human beings (although some reports indicate that the Russians have experimented with high doses of vitamin C as an abortion-inducing agent). Nevertheless, he adds, "although ascorbic acid is a highly valuable and useful vitamin and drug, it is also an exceptionally reactive substance biochemically and should be treated with respect."

Dr. G. N. Schrauzer of the Department of Chemistry at the University of California at San Diego has proposed the theory that an excessive consumption of vitamin C could in fact *lead to* scurvy. "If you impose a stress on the body," Dr. Schrauzer told me, "by giving it an excess of a chemical, that is a shock to the body at first. It sees the excess chemical, in this case vitamin C in high doses, as an intruder. But after a while, the body adjusts by making enzymes to get rid of the excess. But the machinery is nonspecific. When you stop taking the excess vitamin C and take only what you are supposed to, the enzymes are still there. They do not know this is a normal amount of C, and get rid of that too."

Schrauzer, a small man dressed in an open white shirt and baggy pants, is something of an actor. As he talks to me, he smiles like a cat toying with an ingénue mouse. As he throws his feet up on his desk, he grasps his cigarette gingerly between thumb and index finger, places a match gently to the cigarette's tip and draws smoke through it through pursed lips. The procedure finished, he continues talking in his just-this-side-of-Americanization German accent, his words punctuated by hard *v*'s and sibilant *s*'s: "You see, long before all this started, as an experiment I took 10 to 20 grams of vitamin C a day for a few weeks. When I stopped taking these doses, I got scurvy. My body, you see, was getting rid of all the vitamin C."

Two Harvard University nutritionists, Dr. Frederick J. Stare and Dr. K. C. Hayes, have also warned that, theoretically, vitamin C can have detrimental effects. "The large number of people who may be exposed to Pauling's large dosage will probably unveil a percentage of unsuspecting persons who may suffer as-yet-un-known damage, a posssibility that should not be taken lightly by men of science," the duo warns. "For example, it has been well known for many years that vitamin C increases the absorption of iron. Does the same happen with other minerals, including one currently in the news, mercury? If so, the vitamin cultists may be in for some trouble far more serious than a drippy nose."

Some physicians and physiologists shrug off Pauling's theoretical suggestions for the use of vitamin C. The body, they say, will absorb only what it needs anyway—a handful of milligrams—and then just simply flush out the rest. But some experts point out that even if excess C is flushed out of the body, the process by which the C is expelled is anything but innocuous. In order to cope with the excess ascorbic acid and to prepare it for excretion, the body has to find other materials, alkaline products, to neutralize the ascorbic acid. "All of a sudden you dump all this junk into it," says Dr. Kaufman, "and the body doesn't know what the hell is going on. It starts running around like mad pulling everything out so it can neutralize the stuff, and that means the essentials, too, like other minerals. There is all this acid to neutralize and the body will even start using calcium. Calcium salts are slightly insoluble and will precipitate out of the water the kidneys start pumping to get rid of the ascorbic acid. Eventually, you could develop kidney stones."

"If you tell people without a background knowledge of the effects of large doses of vitamin C to go out and take 1,000, 5,000, 10,000 milligrams of vitamin C a day, you are essentially setting up an unethical, uncontrolled experiment with humans to find out what effects these large doses may have," Professor Lutvak says. "The excess has to be excreted, and when people are taking these large quantities, more than 99 percent appears in the urine in the course of a day. They start putting out tremendous quantities of urine because they get very thirsty and drink large quantities of fluids. If they don't drink a proper amount of fluid, the stuff, which is water-soluble but not very soluble, tends to crystallize out in the kidneys and produces damage to the kidneys directly. The other effect, since ascorbic acid is water-soluble, is that by putting large quantities into the gut at once, water is drawn into the colon and produces diarrhea.

"Vitamin C also reacts to all the tests we have for diabetes in the same way as sugar does. We have seen patients who are diabetics or borderline diabetics who have treated themselves with vitamin C and who thought when they tested themselves for sugar that their diabetes was getting worse, who then increased their insulin and put themselves into insulin shock."

Professor Pauling, of course, is not impressed by the theoretical other side of his vitamin C coin. "The claim that patients taking heavy doses of vitamin C develop kidney stones has never been documented," he counters. "I have not been able to find a report in the medical literature of even a single person with kidney stones shown to be caused by ascorbic acid." Vitamin C critics agree that there is no hard-and-fast proof yet that vitamin C leads to kidney stones—but, after all, they ask, if the theoretical good sides can be touted, why not the theoretical bad sides too? And if the theoretical advantages of a regimen must be considered by conventional scientists, the theoretical disadvantages must be taken into consideration by the vitamin enthusiasts. "We know that excessive vitamin C causes the body to form oxalic acid, an ingredient in some kidney stones, especially those associated with gout," Dr. Charles King, one of the pioneer vitamin C researchers, argues. "There is no proof that huge doses of vitamin C can cause the stones to form, but we have no evidence of the effect of the long-term intake at this level—and kidney stones develop slowly."

Two other vitamins—or, rather, the theoretical and unproven administration of massive doses of those vitamins for a variety of human ills—bear additional witness to the proposition that an all-too-enthusiastic embrace of theoretical medicine can blind its practitioners to serious side consequences that may flow from an imperfectly tested supposition. The vitamins in question are vitamins D and A.

Vitamin D's most outstanding achievement has been to eradicate rickets, the disease that for centuries left children with bowed legs, knock knees, swollen joints, and generally distorted and weak arms and legs. Recently, however, vitamin D has been prescribed as a cure for problems ranging from asthma to rheumatoid arthritis, psoriasis, and sarcoidosis, a tubercular illness that often affects many parts of the body, including the liver, the spleen, the eyes, and the small bones of the hands and the feet.

Vitamin D, researchers have found, is a fascinating vitamin. It is manufactured in the body through the combined action of sunlight (or artificial ultraviolet light) and a number of fatty substances within the cholesterol family. Fifteen minutes of sunlight on a patch of skin covering an area no bigger than the nose can provide sufficient vitamin D to prevent rickets and keep children growing well. The importance of sunlight in the formation of vitamin D was apparent even to researchers in the nineteenth century. Although they did not know anything about vitamin D as a chemical entity, they noted that children in the southern, sunny climes of Europe seldom, if ever, suffered from rickets. Only those children in climates marked by long, dark winters, or children growing up in the urbanized areas of the industrial nations where buildings crowded together obliterated the sun completely and where air pollution was an effective barrier to the short ultraviolet rays coming from the sun, developed rickets on a consistent basis. As late as 1926, up to 96 percent of the children in New Haven, Connecticut, suffered to one extent or another from rickets.

Although vitamin D is easily manufactured by the body in the presence of sunlight, it occurs rarely in foods and is present in only a few nutrients, particularly egg yolks and liver (largely fish-liver oils). Nevertheless, the vitamin is powerful. A tablespoon of cod-liver oil, the dose given to children before the vitamin was actually identified, isolated, and manufactured synthetically in less noxious forms, contains only one millionth of an ounce of pure vitamin D. Put another way, vitamin D is so powerful that one ounce of the substance can provide one day's ricket-preventing dose for one million children.

But if the vitamin is powerful it is also treacherous. Many vitamins are water-soluble—that is, they dissolve in water as they are used by the body and are excreted along with excess water as the body cleanses itself every day. But vitamin D dissolves—breaks down—only in fats. Since fat accumulates in the body, excess vitamin D, bound to the fat, stored with the fat in various tissues around the body. As the vitamin accumulates beyond the amounts needed by the body, it brings on a host of devastating occurrences. Vitamin D's function is to help the body retain and utilize enough calcium and phosphorus to help bones develop properly. Without vitamin D, without the minerals the vitamin makes available, bones stay soft. On the other hand, if there is too much vitamin D in the body, the body retains an overly abundant supply of minerals, resulting in a wide assortment of problems. "Many foods are fortified with vitamin D," Professor Lutvak says. "It is present in oleo, butter, milk. So everyone tends to get at least the requirement for D and very often two or three times the requirement and still be on a safe level. You start getting over that and the body starts accumulating it and the toxic effects occur. Blood calcium goes very high, bones start dissolving, bone pain occurs, kidney stones develop, calcification occurs in the blood vessels everywhere in the body, in the heart, the brain, the muscles. It can lead to death in months."

It is difficult to say precisely what constitutes an overdose of vitamin D because various people tolerate the vitamin at various levels. One woman taking doses of vitamin D developed dangerous calcium levels in her bloodstream after only a few weeks. Her husband, taking the same daily dose, developed no problems. Some people who have taken 750,000 international units of vitamin D a day (the Recommended Daily Allowance is 400 international units a day for men, women, and children) have shown signs of vitamin D poisoning after twelve days. Other people who have taken as little as 50,000 international units a day have shown signs of excessive calcification within a few weeks. Some adults have tolerated 500,000 units a day for a year without difficulties. One woman who took more than 112,500,000 (that's right, one hundred and twelve million five hundred thousand) international units of vitamin D over a three-year period on the advice of a friend, who told her that the vitamin would cure her arthritis, developed irreversible kidney failure as a result of her vitamin D overindulgence.

In children, vitamin D poisoning is often evident at substantially lower doses. Although the recommended intake for infants is 400 international units a day, many children actually take in greater amounts because they drink milk fortified with D, they get supplemental vitamin pills loaded with D, and they play outdoors. Thus children who have been fed excessive amounts of the vitamin—by accident or by mothers who believe that massive amounts of the vitamin are essential for good health—have developed severe mental defects, severe kidney damage, overly thick bones at the base of the skull, and dental problems. Dr. Helen Taussig, a prominent children's cardiologist, believes that excessive vitamin D intake could also be responsible for the onset of aortic stenosis, a condition in which the valve between the pumping chamber of the heart and the aorta becomes stiff and grows increasingly incapable of regulating properly the flow of blood to the body. According to Dr. Taussig, researchers have found several children with high levels of vitamin D, a history of high calcium in the blood, or both, who have also been plagued by aortic stenosis.

Vitamin A is yet another vitamin abused because enthusiasts are much too ready to endow it with powers it does not have. Again, the levels at which vitamin A can become toxic—can induce bone and joint pain, fatigue, insomnia, loss of hair, drying and fissuring of the lips, weight loss, symptoms that mimic brain tumors—have not been firmly established. Overdoses of vitamin A can theoretically lead to changes in the liver, the organ where much of the vitamin is stored. However, one man who had taken 5 million international units of vitamin A over the span of a few years did not have liver damage when he died (from causes unrelated to the vitamin). Other people have taken up to 100,000 international units a day for two or three years before they have begun to show some of the symptoms commonly asssociated with vitamin A poisoning. On the other hand, an eighteen-year-old girl who had been taking 50,000 international units of vitamin A in the hope that the vitamin would cure her acne fell into deep depressions, lost her appetite, had trouble sleeping, lost weight, suffered from blurred vision, and stopped having her period six months after she began her regimen. When she began to suffer excruciating headaches as well, her mother checked her into a hospital because a doctor suspected that a brain tumor might be involved. Exhaustive brain studies failed to uncover a malignancy, and when doctors learned of her vitamin A intake, they suggested she stop taking the vitamin. Within two weeks her symptoms disappeared.

It is highly unsettling to think that anyone can practice theoretical medicine who wants to see himself as a savior of mankind, as the imaginative discoverer of an answer to an enigma (heart disease, schizophrenia, senility, the common cold) that has puzzled the keenest of scientific minds. If you don't have to prove your theory beyond a shadow of a doubt before sending millions running off to try it, there is almost no theory you cannot construct, no theory that cannot be used to rationalize the prescription of virtually anything as a new miracle drug. That is especially true when the theory is based on the prescriptions of vitamins, products that already have such a wide acceptance among the general public. Any psychiatrist who has watched many of his mentally ill patients resist other treatments, any doctor who has watched his heart-disease patients die off despite his best attempts to help them, any physician who has had to battle fiercely to win an extra six months of life for a patient, any physician, in fact, who does not want to acknowledge that medical science is limited, that in the face of most catastrophic diseases he has no easy answers, can fall prey to the lures of theoretical medicine, to magnificent, dazzling, but flimsy, theories that allow him (and by extension his patients) escape the often very depressing facts about the state of medical knowledge.

One might be able to make the argument that there is nothing wrong with theoretical medicine, if the physician practicing it were to restrict it to his own patients. Then he could carry on with them the kind of exacting experiments that might induce other researchers to look upon his ideas seriously, to try to confirm and refine them. If he were not willing to carry out such experiments with his own patients (believing the experiments to be immoral), he could go on prescribing the vitamins, and the ethics of prescribing an inadequately tested compound would be strictly between him and his patient (or, of course, between the doctor and the local medical society's committee on quackery). If, applied empirically, the compounds were to prove ineffective or even harmful, the number of affected people, looking at this in the coldest possible terms, would be small. In time, the physician, discredited in his own community, would either have to relinquish his pet theory or would have to leave town.

But because vitamin theoreticians see themselves as the heralds of ideas that will save mankind, they are not content to work out—to prove or disprove—their ideas within the confines of their practices or research situations. Rather, they seek to carry their message directly to millions and millions of people. Publicity, in other words, has been given the same, if not superior, consideration as scientific study. This, in effect, has several consequences. It means that no theory can really be proven or disproven as a result of careful observations of those who submit to its recommendations. Every time a vitamin E theorist or a megavitamin therapist publishes a book or magazine article touting his ideas, millions run out to buy the vitamin. No one really knows precisely what is wrong with the people who stoke themselves with the vitamins and swear by them, how long they take their vitamins, what the effects really are, or how those people really fare in comparison to others who don't take the vitamins. And, if the vitamin, in the final analysis, does not work, there is no way that this negative proof can be of any use. Those disappointed with the results simply disappear into the woodwork, leaving no trace of their negative experience, no way to warn the new hopefuls who, upon reading the latest claims made by a vitamin theorist, are at the moment rushing to the drugstore to stock up on the vitamin, of the futility of the regimen. Of course, since the physicians practicing vitamin therapy address themselves to millions of people, those doctors do not get a proper feedback either. They might see and keep in touch with a score of patients, particularly those who believe they have been helped. But they never see again or hear from again the hundreds who might have come from Portland or Detroit or New Orleans for help, who got their vitamin prescriptions, went home, took the vitamins for six months or a year and found that, when it came to the bottom line, their psychoses or heart disease had not been affected in the least, and who ultimately threw out what vitamin pills were left.

Finally, because vitamin enthusiasts believe in publicity more than they believe in accurate scientific investigation, they use the media to perpetuate their faulty ideas without ever having to face up to the fallacies of their nonsensical theories. They announce to the world that horse manure, which has vast latent traces of vitamin B_{12},[2] liberally rubbed into the scalp will cure, oh, brain tumors. Researchers from the establishment side, under pressure to verify the claims, will run experiments and find that the claim is wrong. The enthusiasts will not retire to their laboratories to rethink their position. Not at all. They will announce to the world that the establishment just wasn't using enough horse manure, or that it didn't use the horse manure long enough, or that it used horse manure from the wrong kinds of horses. The process is never-ending. The vitamin enthusiast, eyes only on his theories, can weave and dodge incessantly, always appealing to the public at large to believe the validity of his ideas. There is no way conventional science can win in this kind of battle. "You just can't kill Santa Claus," Dr. Gladys Emerson, a UCLA nutritionist, says.

Of course, the tears should be shed not for the conventional scientist but for the public, the ultimate loser in this charade. The irresponsible claims being made by the vitamin enthusiasts, and particularly by doctors who should know better, result in pressure to establishment scientists to test the theories being cranked out in favor of vitamins. And, since the claims are never-ending, the experiments that must be conducted to test them correctly are never-ending. One shudders to think of the time, money, and energy wasted over the last thirty years because other researchers have had to test the half-baked ideas turned out by people adept at giving a scientific sheen to their fantasies. All this, of course, is not to say that "establishment" science should ignore vitamins completely. Determined researchers at the University of Pennsylvania's Department of Dermatology, after all, developed a vitamin A derivative, retinoic acid, to cure some types of acne successfully. Researchers at the University of California at Riverside have synthesized a potent form of vitamin D that has proven to be helpful in treating patients suffering serious bone complications brought on by kidney failure. But both of these new vitamin usages were developed after painstaking research and neither involves the wholesale swallowing of the dangerous vitamins. The dose of the vitamin D derivative is strikingly small; in fact, as little as 0.3 of a microgram, one of the

---

[2] Not to laugh. Some primitive tribes have been known to *eat* manure to give them strength. Vitamin B_{12}, in fact, was isolated in part because some researchers noted that animals that eat cowyard dung generally do not suffer from B_{12} deficiency.

researchers, Dr. Jack Coburn, professor of medicine at UCLA and chief of nephrology at Wadsworth Veterans Administration Hospital in West Los Angeles, says, brings about "striking improvement in bone weakening, a deterioration that is one of the most common abnormalities found in uremia." But it is to say that the very least one could expect is that those people who do believe that vitamins have something new to offer should conduct minimal experiments to separate fact from fancy before they rush out to call the world to attention.

CHAPTER X

Is the
Daily Vitamin Necessary?

Every morning as the sun rises over the land, between 50 and 60 million Americans rise to perform a semireligious ritual—to swallow dutifully, almost obsessively, a pill (maybe two) containing a rich allotment of vitamins and minerals.

Biochemists, doctors, psychiatrists, nutritionists have spent a good deal of time arguing whether or not massive doses of some individual vitamins will have a salubrious effect on a wide assortment of catastrophic and not-so-catastrophic diseases. But that is not to say that they have ignored the millions of Americans who spend almost half a billion dollars a year to keep their medicine chests well stocked with supplies of supplemental vitamins to take in relatively moderate doses every morning. The battle to win the minds and hearts of the common, average vitamin-pill-taker has been as intense as any battle fought over nicotinic acid and schizophrenia, or alpha-tocopherol and heart disease.

There are, it almost goes without saying, two opposing sides to this question as well. There are those who tell the American public that it is foolish to gobble all those vitamin pills because American food supplies all the vitamins and minerals needed for good health. And there are those who tell the public it better take its vitamins because every American is virtually a walking collection of vitamin deficiencies.

Many nutritionists are convinced that the strong grip vitamins have on the public imagination is nothing but a matter of semantics. They believe that Americans love their vitamins because the very word *vitamin* carries in it the promise of life, the promise of vitality. The word was fashioned by Casimir Funk, the Polish chemist, in 1912. Funk suggested that those substances effective against four deficiency diseases known at the time—beriberi, pellagra, scurvy, rickets—were obviously necessary for life (*vita*). They belonged, he thought, to a class of compounds known as *amines*. Therefore, he said in a publication in 1912, the substances should be cal'ed *vitamines*. His contention that the antideficiency substances were amines was eventually proven wrong, and the final *e* was dropped. But the implication—vital for life—remained. That same year, cynics suggest, a Japanese chemist named Suzuki was also trying to determine if a specific nutrient deficiency was responsible for beriberi. He found that it was and named the substance, which he had isolated in rice polishings, oryzamin. But Funk beat him into print and it was Funk's baptism for deficiency-preventing substances that stuck. If Suzuki had won out, some ask, would we be taking hundreds of milligrams of other oryzamins, say oryzamin E, as a sure-fire cure for heart disease? Would oryzamins have stuck in our minds as the things to take, without fail, every morning?

Others who question the mania for vitamin supplementation—whether it is taken in milligrams or grams—look upon the entire vitamin craze as a kind of rebellion, a kind of antiestablishment hit-and-run tactic by people too tired to engage in more meaningful protest. Vitamins, says Dr. Reuben Bitensky, associate dean and associate professor in the School of Social Work at Syracuse University, may be very important to the exhausted, middle-class, middle-aged liberal, the man or woman who no longer has the energy to wage the good fights that had been carried on with so much heat and fire in earlier, younger years.

In discussing various problems, frustrations, and disappointments with middle-aged people who attended group-therapy sessions he sponsored, Dr. Bitensky says, he found that vitamins somehow always seemed to intrude into the discussions, particularly when the conversations were being conducted by people who had once marched, organized committees, sponsored meetings, who had, in sum, expended a great deal of energy for various crusades. Many of these people, Dr. Bitensky reports in an article in the *American Journal of Psychiatry,* did not want to lose their image of themselves as warriors in behalf of worthy causes. "This would lower their own self-esteem as well as imperil the adulation of children, relatives and friends," Dr. Bitensky said in reporting the attitudes exhibited by some of the people in the group. "Vitamins offered a way out of this cul-de-sac. Adherence to the vitamin cult was a means of preserving their image of themselves as antiestablishment. Had not Linus Pauling postulated that vitamin C was being attacked as a cure for colds because the pharmaceutical companies had a vested interest in spurious cold remedies? Was not vitamin E being downgraded by the medical profession because of its investment in the perpetuation of the disease?

"This charge against all the medical establishment in the United States was given all the more credence because of the crisis in the delivery in health services and the resistance of the AMA to liberal solutions. Thus the vitamin evangelists would point to the medical profession's reservations about vitamins as one more example in a long history of opposition to progress in medical services for the populace."

Controversies over vitamins, Dr. Bitensky said, provides the old liberal with an almost inexhaustible supply of righteous causes because there is no dearth of villains on the other side. Not only are the pharmaceutical companies and the AMA battling vitamins, but the food industry is always at work refining vitamins out of the foods made available to the public. "The resulting alliance between the vitamin and organic food devotees brought the vitamin cult into confrontation with the medical empire but also with the food industry. Thus a Goliath had been created that would be a worthy adversary of any liberal David.[1]

"In such a conflict the image of the political crusader could be maintained and even strengthened with substantial rewards for one's self concept. But it was crucial to this accomplishment that it involved only a minimal expenditure of energy. By ingesting vitamins one could fight the establishment with the kind of activism that required no more effort than swallowing. Moreover, the greater

---

[1] From the Preface of the first *The Summary* issued in 1949 by the Shute Institute: "We cherish the role of the David of Canadian medicine for we recall that David of old rejected the weighty armour of the day for lesser weapons, his own skill and agility, and the help of God. With these, he slew his Philistine. . . ."

the dosage, the greater the witness to fervent liberalism and anti-establishment sentiments. The liberals in the group had discovered a holy rite comparable to the sacrament of the Eucharist.''

Most nutritionists who think that swallowing a daily vitamin supplement is a waste of time and money, however, do not bother with speculative ventures into semantics and psychology. Americans waste time and money taking supplemental vitamins, they say, out of an unfounded fear that the food they eat does not supply them with the vitamins and minerals they need.

The fears about our food supplies, the Food and Drug Administration says, are widespread. A survey conducted by the FDA revealed that more then 60 million Americans believe that vitamin supplements are absolutely necessary to maintain health. Many Americans—according to the FDA, at least 20 million—believe, erroneously, that a lack of vitamins will cause most illnesses, including cancer. Many more Americans believe that vitamin supplements are necessary because "wise selections of food are not made, meals are not balanced, and too much 'junk food' is consumed. Built-in inadequacies with the food supply are also believed to be serious wide-scale problems: contaminants such as DDT; 'additives' such as preservatives and artificial colors or flavors may be harmful; refining and processing said to rob food of nutritional value. In fact, a very large majority of the population believes that there are problems with the nation's food supply serious enough to constitute threats to health.''

The FDA is not alone in its belief that essentially Americans need not worry about their vitamin intake. "People who eat normal meals, who are not on some crazy diet, don't need vitamin pills," says Professor Lutvak, who is also an endocrinologist and a professor of medicine at UCLA. "The B complex is widely available. It is present in grains. Our base foods are fortified with vitamin B to above optimal levels. Unless you are living in a cellar and never get outdoors, your body normally synthesizes enough vitamin D for its own needs. Many foods are fortified with vitamin D. It is present in oleo, it is present in butter and milk. It is there naturally or has been added. So everybody tends to get at least the requirement for D and very often two or three times the requirement. Vitamin E deficiency has never been produced in any adult of any species, so we really don't know what vitamin E deficiency amounts to.

"If people weren't getting enough vitamins in foods, we'd see a lot of deficiency problems. But we don't."

Processed foods, frozen foods, many experts say, don't lose their vitamin capabilities as is often claimed. Vitamin C, says Dr. Charles Glen King, one of the researchers who helped isolate the vitamin, is fairly stable at room temperature, or even when heated if the vitamin does not come in contact with copper equipment. Fifty to 8o percent of the vitamin, Dr. King says, is retained in cooked, canned, frozen, and freeze-dried food. In fact, says Dr. King, the average intake of vitamin C in the United States has risen from 69 to 117 milligrams a day, largely because of "the increased use of refrigeration, high-quality canned and frozen produce, and less use of copper containing equipment in the preparation of foods."

All in all, say many experts, American food is as rich in vitamins and nutrients as is necessary. "True," says Dr. Virgil O. Wodicka, director of the FDA's Bureau of Foods, "some vitamins are lost in processing, including cooking in the kitchen. You do get some loss in freezing and canning. But if you compare this with foods that are harvested in the same place (as foods that are ultimately frozen or canned) and that are shipped to the same place fresh, the losses during transportation and holding will be as great, especially after cooking, as the losses in canned or frozen foods. I would hazard a guess that if any one of the three would come out third, it would be fresh, unless you are eating them close to the point of harvest."

Even people who don't faithfully eat the so-called basic foods—meats, fruits, vegetables, and dairy products—are not necessarily lacking vitamins, many nutritionists say. "You can't conclude that people who don't get the things that are listed are badly nourished," Dr. Wodicka says. "You can meet your requirements from a variety of foods. The Eskimos get along very well and they never eat salads. Through trial and error, various ethnic groups have arrived at food combinations that meet their nutritional requirements, but the food combinations vary from group to group and you can't conclude that just because someone eats a different food pattern he is badly nourished."

Thus, according to Dr. Wodicka and others, even people who

eat quickie foods, grabbing something on the run at the local fast-eatery, are not necessarily in danger of suffering from a lack of vitamins. "There are a lot of popular ideas about junk food that are just not true," Dr. Wodicka says. "The McDonald people paid for some nutritional analysis of their stuff, and one of the men at McDonald's told me that with two of their hamburgers, an order of french fries, and a milk shake, you get 1,000 calories that are ideally balanced, except that they are a little low on vitamin A." In other words, there is no way not to get your share of vitamins, some nutritionists say. "Even if you are eating a lot of crap, it is hard to avoid eating some foods that are either fortified by law or that are high in these vitamins to begin with so that enough are left over no matter how long they have been sitting around or what the deterioration is," Professor Lutvak says.

Virtually every other debate over vitamins—there is, the debates whether or not nicotinic acid, ascorbic acid, and alpha-tocopherol are the wonder drugs of the 1970s—pits 99 percent of the establishment physicians and nutritionists against small cliques of dissident doctors and nutritionists. But the debate over the role of the daily supplemental vitamin pill pits nutritionist against nutritionist. Thus many experts in the field frankly question whether the American diet and the foods that compose it are all they are cracked up to be.

As far back as 1922 some very respected nutritionists worried that foods in America have their shortcomings. "There has been a strong tendency during the past two decades to 'purify' food products," Walter H. Eddy, a Columbia University nutrition expert, wrote fifty years ago. "The genesis of this tendency is to be found in a highly laudable ambition to force the manufacturer to eliminate impurities and adulterations and provide clean, wholesome, sanitary food. Unfortunately, in attempting to meet this demand on the part of the public, the food manufacturer has sometimes neglected to ask advice from the nutrition expert and the latter has failed to appreciate the need for advice. The net result has been to discover that nature is often a better chemist than man and has a much better knowledge of what man needs in his diet than the chemist. The chemist employed by the manufacturer has, as a result, gone to such a limit in his development of purification methods as to often eliminate the essential nutrients and the result has been foods that will stand analysis for pure nutrients but which will not stand nature's analysis for dietary efficiency.''

Furthermore, many experts point out, since 1922 and especially since World War II there has been a drastic change in the way people eat in the United States. In 1940, for example, the average American ate 142.4 pounds of meat, 139.1 pounds of fruit, and 116.9 pounds of vegetables. In 1968 the same American was eating just about the same amount of meat. But he was eating only 77.3 pounds of fruit and 95.1 pounds of vegetables. According to Dr. Willard A. Krehl, chairman of the Department of Preventive Medicine at Jefferson Medical College in Philadelphia, ''the most significant and steady decrease of all is the use of cereal products, and if we look only at corn and wheat as the major cereals, we see that corn has dropped from 26.8 to 14 pounds per capita per year, while wheat has dropped from 155 pounds per capita to 109 pounds per person in 1968.''

Much of the change in eating habits—a change for the worse—has come about because life patterns have changed in the United States. ''The nature of the daily routine of life has changed for a very large segment of the population and is continuing to change,'' says Dr. Gordon Graham, professor of international health in the School of Hygiene and Public Health at Johns Hopkins University. ''The traditional pattern of eating three well-balanced meals a day in the home is rapidly becoming a thing of the past. This is already true for breakfast for most people, and this does not respect economic or social class. It is strikingly true for lunch. Well over one third of the people in the United States do not eat lunch at home anymore. Some have relatively well-balanced meals wherever they happen to eat lunch, but many others either do not have them available or do not have the time to devote to the consumption of a traditional meal. So they depend more and more on snacks, which are consumed in a hurry because they are convenient to consume.

''The massive urbanization of rural people, the increasing number of women who work, the changing attitudes of women toward housekeeping, the changes in the nature of the family structure, where the elderly members of the family tend more and more to live alone, all these have resulted in a change, in a constantly changing pattern away from the traditional preparation and consumption of three meals in the home, to the extent that now over 50 percent of the meals consumed in the United States are consumed outside the home. The only thing left is dinner, and this is not the ideal way for man to eat.''

Even dinners at home may soon join the list of endangered meals, some experts feel. Says Dr. Neal Miller, associate director of biological research at Hoffmann-LaRoche in Nutley, New Jersey: "People just don't eat rationally, especially with convenience foods available. At my house, if it can't be made in twenty minutes, forget it. Social activity makes the idea of a balanced diet at home unrealistic. It means everyone should eat a balanced diet whenever they eat. So everyone says, I've got no time today, I'll do it tomorrow.''

That people do not eat balanced diets becomes especially apparent when specific groups of people are studied, many nutritionists say. It is very clear that the elderly, many of whom are poor, many of whom are crippled and limited in their ability to go to the supermarket and to cook, cannot be counted among those people eating three "square" meals a day. "The position of the Council on Foods and Nutrition of the American Medical Association," says Dr. Alan D. Whanger of the Duke University Medical Center, "is that an adequate diet can supply all the nutrients essential for the maintenance of health in normal individuals. One cannot quibble with this except to ask how normal are the elderly as a group in light of the high incidence of chronic illness. According to a U.S. government report, 43 percent of persons over sixty-five have some limitation of activity owing to chronic disability and 86 percent have at least one chronic disease. A good diet is relatively expensive and about a third of elderly persons are poor.''

Nor can it be said that the millions of persons who are constantly on one diet or another are choosing diets that are just brimming with vitamins, nutritionists argue. Unfortunately when many people—including men who diet to trim their waistlines or to cut down their saturated fat intake—diet, they often sacrifice the very foods that are richest in vitamins and other nutrients. It might be said, in fact, that people on diets are getting a marginal supply of vitamins. "An estimated thirty percent of the population is overweight," says Dr. Robert Olson. "In the weight-reducing groups, there are a great number of people who are on calorie-restricted diets. Many women subsist on diets of 1,200 to 1,500 calories, on which it is virtually impossible to meet the RDA for iron and extremely difficult for other vitamins and minerals. If they cut down even further to 1,000 calories or even 800 calories as some do, their diets will not meet the RDA in minerals and vitamins.''

Teen-agers are also among the people who defy the premise that adequate diets can be counted upon to supply the vitamins the body needs. "In looking through the numerous nutrition surveys in this country that have been published,'' Dr. Krehl says, "it is quite evident that breakfast is a meal that is very commonly omitted in the dietary schedule, particularly in the adolescent age groups. It is evident that when this is done, substantial alterations in the pattern of food intake may result. This is particularly true with regard to nutrients commonly ingested at breakfast time and primarily foods that contain vitamin C.'' And away from home, teen-agers do no better choosing food wisely. "Our experience with junior high school children shows that they had no understanding of protective foods, of what foods they should choose,'' one nutritionist who has surveyed teen-age eating habits says. "If they had a dime in their pockets, they did not buy a glass of milk, they would buy a candy bar or a box of sour balls, which are really just all sugar.''

If, as many nutritionists say, it is impossible to escape the conclusion that most people do not choose well-balanced diets, that they allow considerations that have nothing to do with good nutrition—time, personal appearance, tastes—influence their choice of foods; if people are not eating the ideal three-meal-a-day balanced diet that many other nutritionists like to imagine most Americans are eating, what, then, are the chances that they are getting enough vitamins in the foods they eat? The chances seem to be small to nonexistent.

There is, in fact, actually little reason to speculate about what the departure from traditional eating patterns has done to the vitamin and mineral intake of the average American. Many experts point out that the decreased consumption of whole-grain cereal products has had a marked impact on the intake of many vitamins. "As a result of the decrease in consumption of whole-grain cereals, I believe that we can safely say that there has been a decrease in the consumption of vitamin B_6, E, and thiamine,'' Dr. Gladys Emerson, professor of nutrition at UCLA told an FDA hearing on vitamins. In fact, any number of surveys have shown that generally changed eating habits have reduced vitamin intake in virtually every sector of the population. Recently the U.S. Department of Agriculture sponsored 178 studies that analyzed the vitamin status of 12,000 persons. According to Agnes Fay Morgan, a nutritionist at the University of California at Berkeley, the studies indicated that 30 percent of the people surveyed—people ranging in age from five to eighty—had less than two thirds of the amount of ascorbic acid suggested by the Nutrition Board of the National Academy of Sciences–National Research Council. At least 20 percent of the adolescent girls and older women came up short in blood tests for vitamin B complex. Between 15 and 25 percent of all persons surveyed (and about 40 percent of the women over thirty in particular) were low in vitamin A. "In the last few years there has been extensive documentation demonstrating that the diets of 50 percent of the households surveyed could not be considered adequate in providing the Recommended Daily Allowance [2] of important vitamins and minerals," Dr. Graham summarizes. "A large series of surveys carried out in different parts of the country [document] the existence of biochemical and clinical evidence of malnutrition, not limited to our poor, but extending throughout the whole population."

These studies have been conducted not just in broad sectors of the population but among some very specific age groups as well. According to researchers at the National Institute of Child Health and Development's Gerentology Research Center, older people—including elderly persons who live in affluent communities and who have access to good diets—have low B_1, B_2, and B_6 blood levels. A study conducted among teen-agers in Iowa disclosed that they have vitamin shortages. Under ideal conditions, teen-agers (in fact, everybody) would get 60 percent of their vitamin C in their breakfast foods. But many of the teen-agers surveyed skipped breakfast, and thus their only source of vitamin C. "Vitamin C," Dr. Krehl says, "is not abundantly available in a wide enough variety of commonly available foods. The overwhelming majority of nutritional

---

[2] The amount used to be known as the Minimum Daily Requirement. But that term was dropped recently because it was thought to be inadequate. A new term, Recommended Daily Allowance, which implies not a minimum required but an amount needed for general good health (in the opinion of the NRC) was adopted as a substitute.

surveys on populations indicate low intakes of vitamin C, and often this is correlated with improper selection or omission of fresh fruits and vegetables and omission of breakfast.''

While some nutritionists have studied the intake of vitamins among various people, other have studied the specific vitamins that are or are not available to them, that is, they have tried to determine just how much of any given vitamin persons might get even if they do eat everything nutritionists recommend. In 1968, after considerable debate, the National Research Council suggested adults should have a daily intake of 30 international units of vitamin E. Yet various researchers have analyzed the amount of vitamin E available in the diets most people eat and have found that most of these diets are sorely deficient in this particular nutrient. One researcher studied eight typical breakfasts, lunches, and dinners (assuming a by now mythical American who would sit down and eat them) and found that the menus contained an average of 7.4 international units of vitamin E. Some typical menus contained as little as 2.6 international units of E. The menus richest in vitamin E contained 15.4 international units—almost half the Recommended Daily Allowance. Another study, broader in that it measured vitamin E content of sixty different diets, found that 80 percent of them contained less than 5 international units of vitamin E.

This whole business of assuming that Americans receive enough vitamins because of the surfeit of food available to them is, on the whole, a risky assumption to make. In the first place, many nutritionists base their assumptions that the average American gets all the vitamins he needs on the basis of reports detailing what kind of foods are bought in stores. But just because food is bought does not mean, even in these days of high prices, that everyone will eat that food. Some of it may go to waste. Some of it may be eaten by just one member of the family. "Food," says Dr. Krehl, "does not provide nutrition until it passes the teeth, is swallowed, and is made available by the metabolic machinery."

Furthermore, whether some nutritionists want to admit it or not, processed food, which is the mainstay of the American diet, does not give Americans all the vitamins they need. "The influx of new foods and convenience foods, including premixes, TV dinners, and foreign foods, when added to the decreased intake of certain foods, raises serious questions as to whether foods that will be selected and consumed will supply adequate amounts of vitamins and minerals for all segments of the population,'' Dr. Emerson told the FDA. It is true, for example, that the potato, as it comes out of the ground, is very rich in vitamins, particularly thiamine, B_1. And it is true, that the potato, adequately prepared, will give the one who eats it a considerable portion of those vitamins. But millions of households in this country routinely eat potato dishes whipped up out of dehydrated potatoes. Dehydrated potatoes have been processed (obviously) and one of the steps in the processing is the addition of bisulphate, which prevents the potato from turning black in the package as time goes by. But bisulphate is also a thiamine antagonist: it destroys thiamine. Thus it is obviously foolish to attribute to the dehydrated potato the same vitamin qualities that might be attributed to a potato right out of the potato patch.

Dr. Henry Schroeder, emeritus professor of physiology at Dartmouth University Medical School, found that the vitamin B_6 content of foods diminishes during processing. In samples of food he studied, he found that canned seafood has 48.9 percent less B_6 than fresh seafood; that some canned meats have 42.6 percent less B_6 than fresh meat; that canned vegetables have 57 to 77 percent less B_6 than their fresh counterparts; that frozen vegetables have 56 percent less B_6 than vegetables right off the farm. There were similar losses in another B vitamin, pantothenic acid. Canned vegetables lost 46 to 78 percent of the vitamin. Canned meats and other vegetable products lost up to 35 percent of the vitamin, frozen vegetables lost up to 57 percent of their pantothenic acid, and frozen animal products, up to 70 percent.

It might be argued that, even though these products had lost considerable amounts of B_6 and pantothenic acid, there was enough left over to provide an adequate amount for the body to use. Dr. Schroeder found, however, that the vitamin amounts were indeed below adequate levels. ''In respect to vitamin B_6,'' he reported, ''almost all corn, rice, rye, and wheat products had lower concentrations than the required level, as did all canned vegetables and potatoes, all fresh and canned fruits except fresh bananas, all dairy products, and seven of eleven canned meats.'' Amounts of pantothenic acid necessary to provide required amounts of the vitamin, Schroeder reported, were ''not reached in three of four canned dairy products, any canned root vegetable, legumes, and green vegetables, and any frozen vegetable but cauliflower. Levels were adequate in dried and canned fish, but not in all meats. They were adequate in some meats, cornmeal, whole rice, whole rye, oatmeal, bulgur, whole wheat, germ and bran products. Therefore, a diet without whole grains and some meats would supply insufficient pantothenic acid.''

The question whether or not our food intake supplies us with enough vitamins may, in a sense, be premature: the dust from another battle within the nutrition community—what are the best vitamin dosages, what constitutes an adequate level of any given vitamin—has not completely settled.

Some nutrition ''conservatives'' argue that only a minimal intake of vitamins—perhaps even less than the dosages currently recommended by the National Research Council—are really necessary. ''Excessive amounts beyond those required to reverse a vitamin deficiency don't do any good,'' Professor Jukes told me when I talked to him. ''One interesting example of that is in the feed industry. Vitamin deficiencies used to be very common in farm animals and when vitamins were discovered and synthesized, they were put in feeds. The people who make feeds put just enough in there to do the job and if animals would benefit by higher levels, they would put them in because vitamins are very cheap. But they don't. They put in just what the animals need.''

Others, however, argue that far more is necessary, that vitamins in amounts two or three (perhaps even more) times greater than the amount needed to prevent deficiency diseases are necessary. ''Our basic theory,'' says Dr. Bacon Field Chow, professor of biochemistry at the School of Hygiene and Public Health at Johns Hopkins University, ''which has been confirmed by animal experiments and the study of metabolic disease in humans, is that the intake of nutrients at levels which are sufficient to prevent the development of classical deficiency diseases can still present serious metabolic problems that adversely affect human performance. Our laboratory experiments leave no doubt that significant manifestations of marginal deficiencies include decreased learning capability, decreased emotionality, and abnormal social behavior. It is my opinion that man too is affected in the same way by marginal deficiencies in nutrients.'' When mice are fed two or three times the amount of vitamins needed to prevent deficiencies, says Dr. Borsook, of the

University of California at Berkeley, they grow a little larger. But more important, he says, "on an otherwise good diet two or three times the amount of vitamins will delay the onset of senility, even though the animals do not live any longer."

According to many researchers, there is ample proof that generous quantities of vitamins achieve results beyond the mere protection against deficiency diseases. In Japan, says Dr. Horwitt, young people today are two to four inches taller than the previous generation. "In the previous generation," Dr. Horwitt, the man who first defined vitamin E needs, adds, "the Japanese were not sick, as determined by normal medical techniques of examination. In fact, the Japanese have excellent public health practices. The change has been largely an increase in protein and riboflavin consumptions and in the general vitamin supplementation of a larger portion of the population. This increased growth rate shows that you can have nutritional improvement of a population even beyond the concept of correcting obvious nutritional disease. Improving the health of the Japanese by improving their nutrition has increased their growth rate to the point where we now wonder whether their genetic potential for growth is statistically much different from persons of European stock."

(The doubters argue the point. They believe that the spurt in the growth rates of the Japanese can be attributed exclusively to the increased consumption of animal protein among the Japanese since World War II.)

Although there is a good deal of agreement in principle that vitamins in amounts larger than those needed to prevent or cure deficiencies are necessary for optimal health, there is little agreement about where those higher levels should be set. Some researchers, serious and respected nutritionists, feel that the optimal intake of vitamin E should be 30 milligrams a day. But because food analyses have shown that most diets do not yield more than 15 or so international units of vitamin E a day, some researchers have suggested not that people should seek small additional amounts of vitamin E but that the RDA for vitamin E is slipped back to 15 international units. The National Research Council followed these suggestions and cut back its RDA recommendations for vitamin E to about 15 milligrams a day.

As much as conventional nutritionists like to paper over their differences, it is very apparent that there is considerable disagreement within the nutrition community about vitamin E. Almost everybody knows that vitamin E is necessary to protect the polyunsaturated fats in the body. But do we get enough vitamin E to protect all of the additional polyunsaturated fats (PUFFA's as they are affectionately known) we eat these days to protect ourselves against heart disease? Dr. Robert Hodges and Dr. Roslyn Alfin-Slater, a nutritionist at UCLA, write that there isn't much to worry about because "fortunately most of the natural sources of polyunsaturated fatty acids are also excellent sources of vitamin E." *Consumer Reports,* warning its readers against some of the unreasonable claims made in favor of vitamin E, has told its audience that there is plenty of E available to protect against all the PUFFA's we want to eat. Margarine, the magazine told its readers, has thirteen times more vitamin E than butter, and a salmon steak has ten times more vitamin E "than beefsteak, pound for pound."

Others, however, are not so sanguine. Many biochemists point out that vitamin E is perhaps one of the vitamins that is hardest for the body to absorb. Some very respected nutritionists point out that the body may absorb no more than 10 percent of the vitamin E ingested. Others believe that *Consumer Reports* is not being quite accurate (or perhaps its medical advisers are not) in pointing out that E is abundant in margarine. Tests of margarine samples have shown that the vitamin E content among them can vary twenty fold. So getting enough vitamin E from your margarine will depend on what margarine you eat. Biochemists also point out that man requires about 0.6 milligrams of alpha-tocopherol to cover every gram of PUFFA. But only cottonseed oil has the required amount of E to cover its PUFFA's. Corn oil has only 0.36 milligrams of E for every gram of PUFFA, safflower oil, 0.45 milligrams of E per gram of PUFFA, soybean oil 0.28 milligrams of E to every PUFFA gram. Thus, unless a person who eats a good deal of PUFFA's takes care to obtain additional supplies of E, some nutritionists feel, a detrimental PUFFA/E balance could conceivably occur. "The possibility cannot be ignored," says Dr. David C. Herting, a vitamin E researcher with Eastman-Kodak, "that an appreciable increase in consumption of [polyunsaturated oils], whether as supplemental or replacement fat, could result in gradual depletion and eventual deficiency of vitamin E." Adds Dr. Horwitt, "I'm not happy with the lowering of the RDA for E. I think someone pulled a boner."

Nor is there a nailed-down agreement yet on how much vitamin C is really necessary to help a human being maintain optimal health. For years the British Medical Association's Committee on Nutrition pegged its recommended ascorbic acid intake at 30 milligrams a day. Recently it upped the figure to 40 milligrams. The National Research Council in this country now recommends that adults take about 60 milligrams of vitamin C a day—a slight drop from the 70 milligrams a day the council had recommended in 1968. The 60 milligrams for adults (actually, the recommended level varies a bit: it is 80 milligrams for adolescents, 100 for pregnant and lactating women), the NRC believes, provides "added protections against scurvy, promotes wound healing, preserves enzyme activity, favors cellular proliferation, and increases the resistance to common stresses such as those induced by bacterial toxins, low temperature and fatigue." But other nutritionists believe that a vitamin C intake as high as 200 milligrams might be called for. "For optimum health," advocates Dr. Charles Glen King, "I would recommend 100 to 200 milligrams. Some people seem to need more vitamin C than others, and there may be times when a person can use more than he would ordinarily require."

Faced by all of these contradictory ideas and opinions, what should the average American do? From what I have heard and read, I think that three things might safely be said. One is that vitamin supplements are probably in order for a good many people, including teen-agers, preschoolers, poor people, the elderly, people on low-calorie diets, single people who eat most of their meals in restaurants (that sounds like just about everyone in the country!). It can also be said that it is not necessary to spend a fortune on vitamin supplements—a good one does not have to cost more than one to three cents a pill. And, finally, that it is not necessary to take a vitamin pill *every* day. Some vitamins are used up by the body every day. But many are used slowly and are stored in the body for long periods of time. A good intake of B_1 will stay in the body three or four days. The body's supply of vitamin E can last for several months. Ample supplies of other vitamins are kept in the body for a year or more. Thus, depending on one's eating habits, no more than one vitamin pill every other day or so is necessary.

Basically, however, it is not very satisfying to say that people should have some sort of a vitamin supplement. In the first place, encouraging people to use vitamin pills in *any quantity* is not a very good idea because there is the very real possibility that all too many people will, given any encouragement, pop their vitamin pill every morning and then feel—unjustifiably—secure as they move through the rest of the day eating nothing but "empty" calories. They will, in other words, deny themselves other important nutrients just because they have taken their vitamins for the day. In the second place, there is the very good possibility that encouraging people to take vitamins exposes them to potential financial exploitation. Anyone buying vitamins is tempted to drift away from the simple vitamin supplement, the cheap bottle of capsules, to the more expensive and exotic mixtures on the shelf. (The argument made by the vitamin enthusiasts notwithstanding—that pharmaceutical companies oppose vitamins because they are cheap—the vitamin-pill market has proven to be a windfall for the drug companies. In the days when the state of one's vitamin levels was a personal matter and not a part of a national fad, vitamins provided the pharmaceutical companies with modest side incomes. But as economics in the vitamin industry stand today, there is virtually no limit to the benefits vitamins can confer on the financial health of vitamin manufacturers. Between 1965 and 1970 the retail value of vitamin-concentrate sales in the United States rose by $50 million. Between 1966 and 1970 the dollar sales of vitamin E alone rose by 60 percent. When the Food and Drug Administration began to look into the possibilities of limiting the sale of vitamin pills in high dosages and to place other restraints on the sale of the substances, the nation's pharmaceutical companies screamed louder than the most avid vitamin swallowers. "There is a lot of money in vitamins," says Dr. Kaufman. "The companies that turn this stuff out sure as hell don't want their money cut off. Companies like Pfizer, Eastman-Kodak, Hoffmann-LaRoche make carloads of the stuff. If they couldn't make people eat it by the pound, there would be a tremendous loss. When it was decided that vitamin E was a lot of baloney, some of the major manufacturers of E, had their lobbyists down here in Washington in droves trying to convince the Research Council that E was absolutely necessary.")

One logical answer to the vitamin dilemma might be a massive new program to educate both physicians and the public about good, basic nutrition, how to eat well and how to avoid having to take vitamin pills. Physicians, it seems, are particularly ignorant about nutrition. "When we nutritionists talk, we say vitamin supplements are not necessary if you eat the four basic foods," [3] UCLA's Dr. Roslyn Alfin-Slater says. "Now the story is, how do you know what food belongs to each group? Well, because doctors are supposed to be fonts of wisdom, the California Dairy Council queried four hundred doctors and asked them to list what they thought were the four basic foods. The common answers were carbohydrates, fats, proteins, and vitamins!" The number of physicians who can advise their patients properly on how to eat well, agrees Dr. Horwitt, is "fantastically small." "I don't know what the number is, one thousand or two thousand," he adds. "But it might represent no more than one physician out of a hundred. That is particularly true of the younger physicians who were educated in an era when nutrition learning almost disappeared from our medical schools. It's not because of any lack of desire of the young physician to learn more about it. It is just that the curricula of the medical schools has expanded so fantastically over the past twenty years that nutrition is one of the things they sort of ask the physician to go out and learn for himself."

Giving the lay public a new understanding of nutrition may be especially important in view of the confusing array of foods available in supermarkets today. With the wide variety of cans that are opened, packages that are thawed out, cartons that are unwrapped

---

[3] Nutrition education has always been reduced to teaching students—be they high school students suffering through a home economics class or medical students putting up with a quick course on nutrition—about "basic" groups of food. Once it was the "Basic Seven." Now it seems to be the "Basic Four": Fruits, vegetables, meats, and dairy products. However, many nutritionists complain that this penchant for categorizing food is essentially misleading and does not really teach people how to eat well. Many people believe, these nutritionists point out, that eating one representative of each of a "basic" group a day will satisfy the day's requirement for that particular food. And nothing could be further from the truth. For example, many people feel they can satisfy their fruit requirement by eating one type of fruit. But someone eating just one or two bananas will get plenty of potassium but no vitamin C to speak of. Someone gulping down oranges all day will have a good supply of vitamin C but little or nothing of the other vitamins and minerals other fruits can offer. The point of nutritional education should be, experts say, to teach people how to choose a full and healthy diet without resorting to oversimplifications that in themselves can lead to an inadequate diet. Unfortunately, no one knows just quite how to do that.

in order to make the average American meal, a homemaker would need a degree in nutrition and two hours of free time every day to calculate who in the family is eating what foods and getting which vitamins and nutrients. It would be hard to do if the family always ate at home. But since family members eat many meals outside the home (not to mention snacks), the job becomes impossible. Dr. Paul LaChance, professor of nutritional physiology at Rutgers University, estimates that when one takes into consideration meals eaten away from home, snacks eaten during television viewing, before bed, after school, it might not be far off the mark to estimate that many people in this country eat twenty times a day. "There is no convenient way to connect the nutritional knowledge a homemaker has to this eating pattern," LaChance says. "Most nutrition education is based on the traditional eating patterns and certain categories of food, the basic four, for example. The housewife is at a total loss in how to meet nutritional needs in the reality of today's individualized eating patterns with foods that will fit these patterns."

Unfortunately, educating professionals and the public about proper nutrition is no simple matter. Not because doctors don't want to learn or because busy executive women who depend on frozen dinners don't want to listen. But because the field of nutrition education has been flooded in recent years by "nutritionists" whose knowledge of food, proper diets, and vitamins is of dubious value.

A conventional undergraduate degree in nutrition and dietetics—that is, one awarded by major universities—takes four years to complete and includes many courses in general and advanced chemistry, biology, biochemistry, microbiology, human physiology, cultural aspects of nutrition, food chemistry, human nutrition, clinical nutrition, pathology, clinical medicine, sociology, anthropology, psychology and statistics, general dietetics, therapeutic dietetics, community nutrition. A true master's degree program will require the would-be nutritionist to go on for another year and deepen his or her knowledge of these and other fields and, usually, to write a thesis. A doctoral program is even more intense, usually requiring an additional three years of study, oral examinations, and the writing of an extensive thesis the Ph.D. candidate will have to defend against the questioning of his professors.

The nutritionist who earns these degrees, in other words, has a deep and extensive understanding of nutrition and its role in human life.

But all that work and study is too much for many people— especially those anxious to take advantage of a public that often wants quick and easy answers to its nutrition questions. For those men and women not willing to put up with the rigors of a conventional and demanding academic education, there are alternative nutrition "colleges" and "universities." These institutions award B.A.'s, M.A.'s and even Ph.D.'s to students who have shelled out a few thousand dollars and who have read a few books of dubious value—books often written by the director of the school or books whose most distinguishing characteristic is the fact that they survived for a few weeks on a best-seller list. A student at one such institution can earn his "B.A." (or B.S.) in less than a year and his "M.A." (or M.S.) and "Ph.D." in less than nine months. And he can then go out and tell the world that he is qualified to give advice about nutrition.

If the "nutritionists" who gain their degrees at diploma mills were to ply their trade only in little health food stores, the damage they do to the public's understanding of proper nutrition would be minimal. But because many employers never bother to probe the alleged value of an academic degree, hundreds of these false prophets find their way into respectable positions, often acting as nutrition consultants to dentists, physicians, schools, and even governmental agencies. "Even the largest county [Los Angeles] in California recently hired a nutritionist for the County Department of Health Services based on the belief that the applicant had a bona fide B.S. degree in nutrition," the nutrition faculty of the University of California at Davis complained in a 1980 letter to state education officials. "The applicant's 'degree' was from a nonaccredited organization."

The confusion phony nutritionists cause is magnified further by the media. Television shows, often legitimately interested in educating the public, often feature discussions on diet and nutrition. In the hurly-burly world of television, show hosts and producers are too busy to look too deeply into the qualifications of their guests. If someone is available who sports an M.S. or a

Ph.D. after their name, the people who book guests onto the shows assume that the degree is legitimate. As a result, all too often the nutritionists who get on the air are graduates of suspect institutions—people who have phony degrees and who dispense foolish information. The print media have made the same mistake. National publications, including *Us* and *People,* have featured breathless articles about nutritionists without ever bothering to examine whether the credentials held forth by the subjects of their adoration are worthy and credible.

The problem, of course, is not just that the advice dispensed by the graduates of quickie universities is faulty or shallow. It is that the advice will often be downright wrong, misleading, and dangerous. The "nutritionist" who has received his education in an institution dedicated to fast degrees is also likely to be one who will advise that massive doses of vitamins will protect against or cure major ills. One governmental agency sent one of its women agents to a California health-food store that was run by a "nutritionist" who allegedly held the degree of "bachelor of therapeutic science." She told him that she was suffering from breast cancer (she was not, of course) and he promptly prescribed a regimen of vitamins, minerals, and herbal teas. Another agent who went to the nutritionist with a fabricated medical history of emphysema and heart disease was told that she could also be cured by vitamins, minerals, and assorted herbs. The alleged nutritionist eventually left food retailing and opened a school that awards "degrees" in nutrition.

Some nutritionists, however, believe that even if the public were to be exposed only to factual nutritional information, little of it would really sink in. "During World War II, I was chief of Industrial Feeding in the the War Food Administration, where we were dealing with mass education programs," says Dr. Robert S. Goodhart. "Since that time, since 1946, I have been active on individual nutrition-education programs with patients in nutrition clinics. I have the impression both from these programs and from contact with nutritionists in New York—I have been chairman of the Food and Nutrition Council in New York on two occasions and president once—that generally nutrition programs are quite ineffective, whether applied to an individual or through community and mass methods." Education, agrees Dr. Myron Brin, formerly a Harvard University and University of California at Davis nutrition researcher and now assistant director of biochemistry-nutrition at Hoffmann-LaRoche, won't be of much help. "People will go on eating what they want to eat," he says. "Second to cost, personal gratification is the most important factor in choosing food. If you go to a restaurant, you order what you like, not what is nutritionally adequate."

But then, it may not be precisely right to say that educational programs will or will not work. Health and food faddists, after all, have managed to get their points across to millions of people who turn a deaf ear to conventional nutrition experts. Thus it may in fact be more accurate to say that educational programs carried out by more conventional, establishment nutritionists are the ones that will not take hold. And for good reason. By now, most Americans understand that their diets and their way of approaching food do leave something to be desired. They want help. But when the average American does ask for advice—by writing to lay health magazines, newspaper columnists, by calling phone-in radio shows—the establishment nutritionists listen to the question with a blank stare on their faces and then mumble the old stand-by answer about the four basic foods—the very thing already befuddling the petitioner.

The basic problem is that most nutritionists are determined to protect attitudes, ideas, and answers that are consistent with the state of nutrition in this country thirty-five to forty years ago. Deep down inside, most nutritionists know that America, Americans, and food have changed since World War II. But they are afraid to let on, they are scared to voice public doubts about the state of nutrition in America today because to do so, they think, would mean opening a crack in the facade of scientific opposition to quackery that would allow the eat-alfalfa-and-live-to-be-103 crowd to come rushing into the inner sanctum of science, screaming triumphantly, "See, it's what we've been trying to tell you for years." To admit doubt publicly would be to give the vitamin faddists credence in the public mind.

The determination to hold the line against the vitamin faddists by espousing a never-changing faith in the good diets Americans allegedly eat cannot be underestimated. Almost every nutritionist I talked to would not admit that the vitamin intake in the United States was anything but adequate, no ands, ifs, or buts about it. The anxiety with which nutritionists guard against giving an inch of ground to the faddists in public is exemplified best by my interview with Dr. Gladys Emerson while she was still professor of nutrition at UCLA. I knew when I talked with her that she had been much in demand for various and assorted committees on nutrition. Back in 1975 during our nearly two-hour interview, which ranged over the whole field of vitamins, Dr. Emerson steadfastly and staunchly fought off even the slightest suggestion that vitamins in supplemental form were necessary in any way. "I am seventy years old," she told me at the time, "and I am still active. I have never missed a day of school or work since I was seven years old and I don't get vitamins from anywhere except the food I eat. In fact, the only time I have ever taken vitamins in my life was during a short trip to India." Yet, in testimony given to the Food and Drug Administration during its hearings on the new rules it drafted to regulate vitamin consumption, Dr. Emerson cast considerable doubt on the agency's determination to restrict the sale of vitamins and on its contention that vitamin pills are not necessary because the nutrients are widely available in the food we eat. During the hearings, she specifically speculated that vitamin E intake should be optimized because Americans are eating more polyunsaturated fats. And she told the FDA that from a nutritionist's point of view the statement (made by the FDA) that food supplies ample amounts of vitamins is "simply meaningless" and that changed eating habits in the United States "raise certain questions . . . whether . . . foods that will be selected and consumed will supply adequate amounts of vitamins and minerals for all segments of the population." In other words, it is all right to express doubts to a sleepy bureaucrat holding hearings that will probably go unreported in the press, but it is not all right to raise questions to a journalist who will write for public consumption.

As long as nutritionists—and Dr. Emerson is not by far the only member of her profession guilty of "stonewalling" against vitamin supplements in statements she makes for public consumption while saying something else in official semiprivacy—insist on maintaining attitudes most Americans instinctively know are patently absurd, very little progress will be made toward finding a way of keeping the American public well fed and out of the hands of the faddists. It is fairly obvious that the vitamin enthusiasts have made substantial inroads among the American public. But they have not achieved their successes in a vacuum. They have marched on, gathered allies, disseminated their fallacious ideas because in large part the nutrition community has forfeited the public to them.

Of course, nutritionists and others who have been fighting tirelessly against vitamin quackery believe this judgment to be somewhat too harsh. "I do not believe that 'stonewalling' is a major factor in the scientific community's inability to curb quackery nor do I believe that lack of credibility is a major factor," says Dr. Stephen Barrett. "More than one million people are benefiting financially from the sale of vitamins. Moreover, the vitamin pushers have an inherent propaganda advantage. The concept of 'nutrition' insurance is a very clever argument because it appears to cost only pennies a day to be sure 'you are getting enough.' People believe what they hear the most."

Index